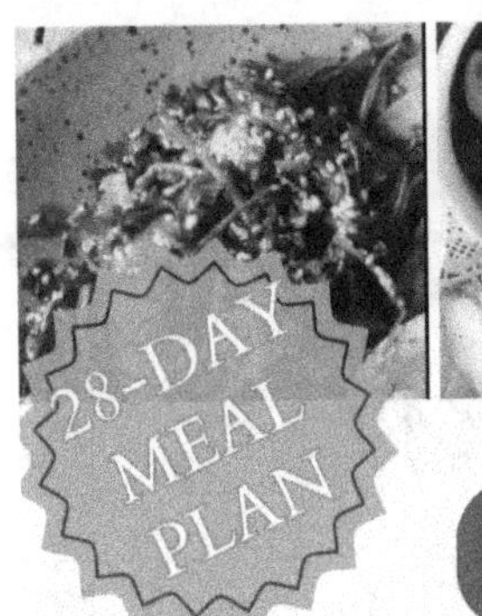

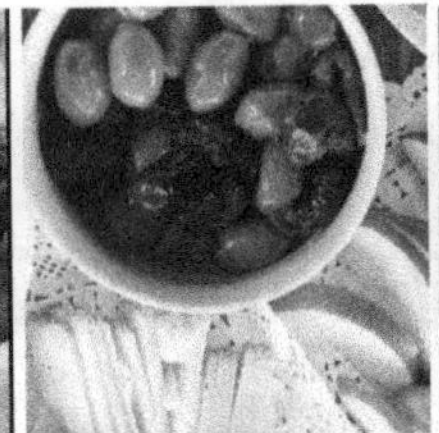

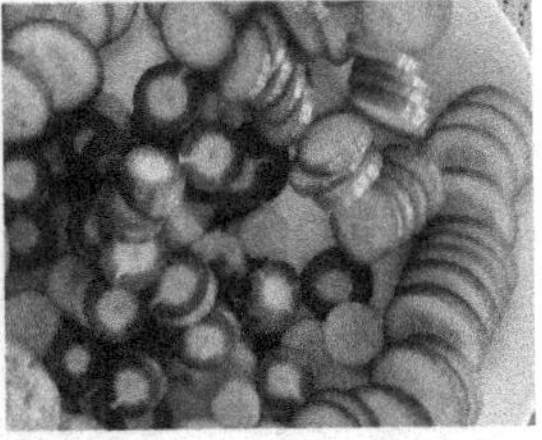

28 DAY

DASH DIET

COOKBOOK

Lose Weight, Boost Energy and Improve your Heart Health with Quick, Delicious and Easy-to-Follow Recipes in Just 4 weeks!

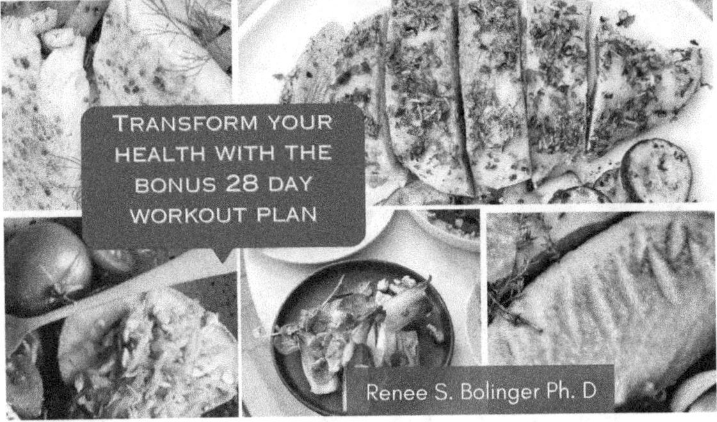

28 DAY DASH DIET COOKBOOK

Lose Weight, Boost Energy and Improve your Heart Health with Quick, Delicious and Easy-to-Follow Recipes in Just 4 weeks!

Renee S. Bolinger Ph. D

Table of Contents

INTRODUCTION

The 28-Day Dash Diet Plan is the perfect way to kickstart your health goals and get on the path to better nutrition. Developed by the National Institutes of Health and regarded as one of the "Healthiest" and "Best" Diets, the Dash Diet is a scientifically-backed, heart-healthy plan that focuses on portion control and encourages the consumption of healthy, nutrient-dense foods. The plan is based on the Dietary Approaches to Stop Hypertension (DASH) study, which showed that eating foods like fruits, vegetables, whole grains, lean proteins, and low-fat dairy could lower blood pressure. The 28-Day Dash Diet Plan provides a comprehensive guide to help you adopt the DASH diet into your lifestyle.

The plan is tailored to those who are looking to lose weight, maintain a healthy weight, and reduce their risk for developing hypertension, heart diseases, and other chronic conditions. The plan includes weekly meal plans, shopping lists, and delicious recipes that make it easy to follow. You'll also find tips on how to make healthy food choices, as well as guidance on portion control and physical activity. Each day will present you with a carefully curated selection of breakfast, lunch, dinner, and snack recipes that are not only delicious but also simple to prepare. With the 28-Day Dash Diet Plan, you'll be able to make small changes that will have a big impact on your health.

Chapter 1:

What is the DASH Diet?

The DASH diet, or Dietary Approaches to Stop Hypertension, is a nutritional program that aims to reduce hypertension, or high blood pressure, by changing the way people eat. It was first developed by the National Heart, Lung, and Blood Institute (NHLBI) in the United States in the early 1990s and has since become a popular choice for managing hypertension and other cardiovascular diseases.

The DASH diet focuses on eating foods that are low in saturated fat, Fat, and cholesterol, while increasing the intake of fruit, vegetables, whole grains, and low-fat dairy products. It also encourages limiting the intake of sodium, sweets, and added sugars. The goal of the diet is to reduce blood pressure and improve overall health.

The diet is a balanced eating plan that is based on the Dietary Guidelines for Americans. It is designed for people of all ages and provides a variety of options for eating healthy. It includes a variety of food groups, including fruits, vegetables, whole grains, lean proteins, low-fat dairy, nuts, and heart-healthy fats.

To follow the DASH diet, individuals should aim to eat more servings of fruits and vegetables, whole grains, and low-fat dairy products. They should also strive to limit their intake of sodium, sweets, and added sugars. Additionally, it is important to get adequate amounts of calcium, magnesium, and potassium.

It has been found to be effective in reducing blood pressure and improving overall health. Studies have shown that following the DASH diet can lower systolic blood pressure by 6mmHg and diastolic blood pressure by 3-4mmHg. It has also been associated with a decreased risk of stroke, heart attack, and coronary artery disease.

Food Groups Included in the DASH Diet:

The DASH Diet includes five major food groups: fruits, vegetables, grains, low-fat dairy products, and lean proteins.

Fruits and vegetables:
Fruits and vegetables should make up the majority of the diet. They are nutrient-dense and provide essential vitamins and minerals that the body needs to stay healthy. Fruits and vegetables are low in fat and calories and high in fibre, which helps promote satiety and healthy digestion. They are also packed with antioxidants, which help protect the body from disease.

Grains:
Grains are an important part of the DASH Diet because they provide carbohydrates, which are the body's main source of energy. It has been scientifically recommended that people choose whole grains, such as oatmeal, brown rice,

whole-wheat bread, and other whole-grain products, over refined grains, such as white bread and white rice. Whole grains are a good source of fibre, which helps keep the digestive system healthy and can help promote weight loss.

Low-fat dairy products:
Dairy products are a great source of calcium, which is important for strong bones and teeth. Low-fat dairy products, such as skim milk, yoghourt, and cheese, are also a great source of protein.
The DASH Diet heavily recommends that people also limit their intake of full-fat dairy products, such as whole milk and cream, due to their high saturated fat content.

Lean Proteins:
Lean Proteins provide essential amino acids, which are needed for the body to build and repair tissues. Lean proteins, such as poultry, fish, legumes, and nuts, are also high in essential vitamins and minerals. Studies recommends that people limit their intake of red meat, bacon, and processed meats due to their high saturated fat content.

Foods to Avoid

Processed meats: Processed meats, such as hot dogs, bacon, and deli meats, are high in sodium and saturated fat. Eating too much of these foods can raise your blood pressure and increase your risk of heart disease and stroke.

Refined grains: Refined grains, such as white bread and white rice, have been processed and stripped of their nutritional value. They contain fewer vitamins, minerals, and fibre than their whole grain counterparts. Eating too many refined grains can increase your risk of obesity and diabetes.

Sweets and sugary drinks: Sweets and sugary drinks, such as soda and candy, are high in calories and added sugar. Eating too much of these foods can lead to weight gain and an increased risk of obesity and diabetes.

Fried foods: Fried foods, such as french fries, are high in saturated fat and calories. Eating too much of these foods can increase your risk of heart disease, stroke, and obesity.

Alcohol: Alcohol is high in calories and can interfere with weight loss efforts. Drinking alcohol can also increase your blood pressure and the risk of some cancers.

Benefits of the DASH Diet

The DASH diet has been shown to be effective in reducing blood pressure. It also has many other health benefits, including promoting weight loss, reducing risk of stroke, diabetes, and heart disease, and improving cholesterol.

Weight Loss

Following the DASH diet is an excellent way to lose weight. It is based on healthy, whole foods that are low in calories, fat, and sugar. This helps to reduce your overall calorie intake, leading to weight loss. Additionally, because the diet is rich in fibre and protein, it helps to keep you feeling full and satisfied.

Lowering Blood Pressure

The DASH diet was specifically designed to reduce high blood pressure. It includes lots of fruits, vegetables, and whole grains, which are all high in potassium, magnesium, and calcium, which are known to help lower blood pressure. Additionally, the DASH diet limits the intake of sodium also known as salt, which helps to further reduce blood pressure.

Lowering Risk of Stroke

The DASH diet can also help reduce the risk of stroke. Eating a diet rich in fruits, vegetables, and whole grains can help reduce inflammation, which is a common cause of stroke. Also, the DASH diet is low in saturated fat, which can help lower "bad" cholesterol, further reducing the risk of stroke.

Reducing Risk of Diabetes

The diet reduces the risk of type 2 diabetes. Eating a diet rich in fruits, vegetables, and whole grains can help regulate blood sugar levels, reducing the risk of diabetes. Additionally, the DASH diet is low in saturated fat and added sugars, which can help to reduce risk of diabetes as well.

Improving Cholesterol

Eating a diet rich in fruits, vegetables, and whole grains can help increase the amount of "good" cholesterol, while reducing the amount of "bad" cholesterol. The intake of saturated fat and added sugars are limited by the diet which can further reduce "bad" cholesterol.

Chapter 2:

The 28-Day Dash Diet Plan

In this section we will be talking about all you need to know that will help you during the 28-Day Dash Diet Plan

Daily Nutrients Guide

Recommended portions from each food category for a 2,000-calorie DASH diet:

Grains: 6–8 servings each day. A serving can be 1/2 cup cooked cereal, rice, or pasta, 1 slice of bread, or 1 ounce dry cereal.

Vegetables: 4–5 servings each day. One serving is 1 cup raw leafy green vegetables, 1/2 cup cut-up raw or cooked vegetables, or 1/2 cup vegetable juice.

Fruits: 4-5 servings each day. A serving equals one medium fruit, 1/2 cup fresh, frozen, or canned fruit, or 1/2 cup fruit juice.

Low fat Dairy: Consume two to three servings of fat-free or low-fat dairy products each day. One serving equals 1 cup milk or yoghurt, or 1 1/2 ounces cheese.

Lean meats, poultry, and fish: six 1-ounce portions or less each day. One serving equals one ounce of cooked meat, poultry, or fish, or one egg.

Nuts, seeds, dried beans, and peas: 4 to 5 servings per week. One serving equals 2 tablespoons seeds, or 1/2 cup cooked dry beans or peas.

Fats and oils: 2–3 servings per day. One serving equals one teaspoon vegetable oil, one tablespoon mayonnaise,

Sweets and added sugars: 5 or less servings per week. One serving equals 1 tablespoon sugar, jelly or jam or 1 cup lemonade.

Projected daily Nutritional targets for the DASH diet plan:

Sodium: Aim for a daily intake of no more than 2,300 milligrams (mg) of sodium, with an optimal goal of 1,500 mg or less.

Potassium: Encourage a daily consumption of approximately 4,700 mg of potassium-rich foods, such as fruits (e.g., bananas, oranges) and vegetables (e.g., spinach, sweet potatoes).

Calcium: Studies recommend a daily intake of 1,000-1,200 mg of calcium. This can be achieved through consuming low-fat dairy products, fortified plant-based milk alternatives, and calcium-rich foods like leafy greens (e.g., kale) and almonds.

Magnesium: Emphasise a daily consumption of around 320-420 mg of magnesium. Foods like nuts, seeds, whole grains, and leafy greens are good sources of magnesium.

Protein: Aim for about 0.8-1.0 grams of protein per kilogram of body weight per day. Protein accounts for around 18% of calories.

Fibre: The recommended daily intake of fibre is around 25-38 grams, depending on age and gender.

Fats: Aim to keep saturated fat intake below 10% of total daily calories. Fat accounts for around 27% of calories. Saturated fat accounts for 6% or less of total calories.

Carbohydrates: Carbohydrates account for around 55 percent of calories.

Cholesterol: Cholesterol is restricted at 150mg.

Stocking Your Kitchen

Start with Fruits and Vegetables

Fruits and should be your go-to for snacking and adding to meals. You'll want to make sure you have a variety of colors and types, such as:

- Apples, bananas, oranges, and other fresh fruits
- Carrots, celery, bell peppers, tomatoes, and other crunchy vegetables
- Frozen fruits and vegetables for quick and easy meals
- Canned sweet potatoes, squash, and other ready-to-eat items

Include Healthy Grains

Try to consume at least three servings of whole grains daily. Good options include: Brown rice, Quinoa, Whole wheat pasta, Whole wheat bread, Oatmeal, Bulgur, Barley, Farro, Popcorn, Wild rice

Stock Up on Lean Protein
Opt for leaner options such as: Skinless chicken, Fish and seafood, Lean beef and pork, Beans and legumes, Tofu and tempeh, Eggs, Nonfat or low-fat Greek yoghurt, Low-fat cheese, Nuts and nut butters

Low-Fat Dairy: Olive oil, Canola oil, Avocado oil, Coconut oil, Nuts and nut butters, Seeds, Avocados Olives, Fish and seafood, Flaxseeds

Herbs and Spices: Herbs and spices are great for adding flavor to your meals without adding sodium. Try to use fresh herbs and spices like rosemary, garlic, basil, oregano, and cumin when cooking.

Kitchen Utensils and Appliances

Having the necessary utensils and appliances in your kitchen will make your journey through the 28 day dash diet plan easier. The needed utensils and appliances include:

1. Non-Stick Pans: Non-stick pans are essential for cooking on the 28 day dash diet meal plan. You'll want to avoid cooking with oil and butter, so a non-stick pan will help you to prepare healthy meals without having to use extra fat.

2. Griddle: A griddle is a great tool to have in your kitchen, as it allows you to cook multiple items at once. You can use it to make omelettes, pancakes, grilled vegetables and much more.

3. Blender: A blender is a must-have for any kitchen, and it's especially useful for the 28 day dash diet meal plan. You can use it to make smoothies and other healthy drinks, as well as sauces and dressings.

4. Food Processor: A food processor is a great tool for quickly chopping, slicing, and dicing ingredients. It's especially useful for making meals such as soups, stews, and salads.

5. Steamer: A steamer is the perfect tool for making healthy, delicious meals on the 28 day dash diet meal plan. You can use it to steam vegetables, fish, and even grains and beans.

6. Slow Cooker: A slow cooker is an invaluable tool for making low-sodium, low-fat meals. You can use it to make soups, stews, and casseroles with ease.

Meal Prepping Tips

- **Invest in quality containers**: Invest in quality containers for storing your prepped meals. Make sure they're airtight and durable enough to last through the week.

- **Double up:** If you're making a meal that can be frozen, double the recipe and freeze half for a later date. This will save you time in the future and ensure that you always have a healthy, Dash Diet-friendly meal on hand.

- **Plan ahead:** Try to plan ahead for meals by prepping ingredients for multiple dishes. For example, if you're prepping roasted vegetables for one meal, you can use the same vegetables for a salad or stir-fry later in the week.

- **Have fun:** Meal prepping doesn't have to be a chore. Choose recipes that you'll enjoy and make sure to treat yourself to something special once in a while.

Grocery shopping tips

- **Plan ahead**: Planning ahead is key. Make a grocery list of all the ingredients you will need for the week, and shop accordingly. This ensures that you have all the necessary ingredients on hand and can prepare meals quickly and easily.

- **Buy fruits and vegetables in season:** Fruits and vegetables are key components of the Dash Diet and should be included in your grocery list. When possible, buy fruits and vegetables that are in season as this will ensure that you are getting the most nutrient-dense produce.

- **Stock up on pantry staples:** The Dash Diet also includes pantry staples such as canned beans and legumes, whole grains, and nuts and seeds. Make sure to stock up on these items so that you can easily add them to your meals.

- **Buy frozen fruits and vegetables:** Frozen fruits and vegetables are a great way to get your daily servings of fruits and vegetables. Frozen produce is often picked and frozen at its peak ripeness, ensuring that you are getting the most nutrient-dense foods.

- **Get low-fat dairy products:**

- **Get healthy snacks:** Snacking is an important part of the Dash Diet. When grocery shopping, make sure to buy healthy snacks such as nuts, seeds, and fresh fruits and vegetables. These foods can help satisfy your hunger between meals and provide important nutrients.

Portion control

Pre-portion meals: Pre-portioning meals ahead of time is one of the best ways to practice portion control. This can be done by portioning out individual servings of meals into containers or bags, so you can grab and go.

Use smaller dishes: By using smaller plates, bowls, and cups, you'll be able to better control your serving sizes.

Measure ingredients: Measure out foods like grains, proteins, and vegetables to get an accurate idea of how much you should be eating.

Track your intake: Keeping a food diary and recording your meals and snacks can help you get an idea of how much you're actually eating.

Fill half your plate with vegetables: By filling your plate with non-starchy vegetables, you'll be able to better control your portions and ensure you're getting enough nutrients.

Eat slowly: This might sound unbelievable or funny but Eating slowly can help you practice portion control. Take your time when eating and savor your food. This will help you to better recognize when you're full and practice mindful eating.

Utilizing leftovers

With a busy lifestyle, it can be difficult to make time for meal prep every day. That's why it's important to know how to make the most of your leftovers.

- One way to make the most of leftovers is to repurpose them into other meals. For example, you can use leftover cooked vegetables to create a stir fry, or leftover cooked chicken to make a salad. This can help you save time and money on food, as well as help you stick to your DASH diet meal plan.

- Another way to utilize leftovers is to freeze them. Freezing leftovers can help extend their shelf life and make them easier to use later on. Soups, stews, and casseroles can all be frozen and then easily reheated when you need a quick meal. This can help you avoid spending money on unhealthy convenience foods when you're short on time.

- Finally, you can also use leftovers as an ingredient in a completely new dish. For example, you can use leftover cooked vegetables to make a frittata, or leftover cooked chicken to make a soup. This is a great way to get creative with your meals and make something unique and delicious.

Chapter 3:

28-Day Dash Diet Meal Plan

Day 1:
Breakfast: 2 eggs over-easy, 2 slices of whole grain toast, ½ cup of fresh fruit.
Snack: 1 cup of plain Greek yoghurt, ½ cup of almonds.
Lunch: 4-ounce grilled chicken breast, ½ cup of cooked quinoa, 1 cup of steamed vegetables.
Snack: 1 hard-boiled egg, 2 slices of whole wheat toast.
Dinner: 4-ounce salmon fillet, 1 cup of roasted cauliflower, ½ cup of cooked brown rice.

Day 2:
Breakfast: Oatmeal with blueberries and walnuts, 1 cup of skim milk.
Snack: 1 apple, ½ cup of low-fat cottage cheese.
Lunch: Turkey wrap with lettuce, tomato, and avocado, 1 cup of fresh fruit.
Snack: 1 cup of plain Greek yoghurt, ½ cup of almonds.
Dinner: 4-ounce grilled chicken breast, ½ cup of cooked quinoa, 1 cup of steamed vegetables.

Day 3:
Breakfast: Egg white omelette with spinach, mushrooms, and tomatoes, 2 slices of whole grain toast.

Snack: 1 cup of plain Greek yoghurt, ½ cup of almonds.

Lunch: Bean and vegetable soup, 1 slice of whole wheat bread.

Snack: 1 hard-boiled egg, 2 slices of whole wheat toast.

Dinner: 4-ounce grilled salmon fillet, 1 cup of roasted cauliflower, ½ cup of cooked brown rice.

Day 4:

Breakfast: Overnight oats with banana and walnuts, 1 cup of skim milk.

Snack: 1 apple, ½ cup of low-fat cottage cheese.

Lunch: Spinach salad with grilled chicken, 1 cup of fresh fruit.

Snack: 1 cup of plain Greek yoghurt, ½ cup of almonds.

Dinner: 4-ounce grilled chicken breast, ½ cup of cooked quinoa, 1 cup of steamed vegetables.

Day 5:

Breakfast: Smoothie with banana, almond milk, and protein powder.

Snack: 1 cup of plain Greek yoghurt, ½ cup of almonds.

Lunch: Hummus wrap with lettuce, tomato, and cucumber, 1 cup of fresh fruit.

Snack: 1 hard-boiled egg, 2 slices of whole wheat toast.

Dinner: 4-ounce grilled salmon fillet, 1 cup of roasted cauliflower, ½ cup of cooked brown rice.

Day 6:

Breakfast: 2 eggs over-easy, 2 slices of whole grain toast, ½ cup of fresh fruit.

Snack: 1 apple, ½ cup of low-fat cottage cheese.

Lunch: Grilled vegetable wrap with hummus, 1 cup of fresh fruit.

Snack: 1 cup of plain Greek yoghurt, ½ cup of almonds.

Dinner: 4-ounce grilled chicken breast, ½ cup of cooked quinoa, 1 cup of steamed vegetables.

Day 7:

Breakfast: Oatmeal with blueberries and walnuts, 1 cup of skim milk.

Snack: 1 hard-boiled egg, 2 slices of whole wheat toast.

Lunch: Tuna salad sandwich on whole wheat bread, 1 cup of fresh fruit.

Snack: 1 cup of plain Greek yoghurt, ½ cup of almonds.

Dinner: 4-ounce grilled salmon fillet, 1 cup of roasted cauliflower, ½ cup of cooked brown rice.

Grocery Shopping List for WEEK 1

Protein:

- 14 eggs
- 8 ounces of grilled chicken breast
- 8 ounces of salmon fillet
- 1 can of tuna

Dairy/Dairy Alternatives:

- 2 cups of plain Greek yoghurt
- 1 cup of skim milk
- 1/2 cup of low-fat cottage cheese
- Almond milk (for smoothies)

Fruits:
- Fresh fruit (choose a variety of your favorites such as blueberries, bananas, apples)
- 1 cup of blueberries
- 1 cup of sliced apples

Vegetables:
- 1/2 cup of fresh fruit (for breakfast day 1)
- 1 cup of steamed vegetables (for lunch day 1 and dinner day 1)
- 1 cup of roasted cauliflower (for dinner day 1 and dinner day 3)
- 2 cups of spinach (for lunch day 4)
- 1 cup of roasted cauliflower (for dinner day 4)
- 1 cup of steamed vegetables (for dinner day 5)
- 1 cup of roasted cauliflower (for dinner day 5)
- 1 cup of grilled veggies (for lunch day 6)
- 1 cup of steamed vegetables (for dinner day 6)
- 1 cup of roasted cauliflower (for dinner day 6)
- 1 cup of fresh fruit (for lunch day 7)

Grains/Breads:
- 4 slices of whole grain toast
- 1/2 cup of cooked quinoa
- 2 slices of whole wheat toast
- 1 slice of whole wheat bread
- 1/2 cup of cooked brown rice
- Whole wheat wraps/tortillas

Nuts/Seeds:
- 1/2 cup of almonds

- Walnuts

Miscellaneous:
- Bean and vegetable soup (can or homemade)
- Hummus
- Lettuce
- Tomato
- Avocado
- Cucumber
- Protein powder (for smoothies)

Recipes

DAY 1
Breakfast: Egg Toast Fruit

Ingredients:
- 2 eggs
- 2 slices of whole grain toast
- ½ cup of fresh fruit

Instructions:
1. Heat a non-stick pan over medium heat.
2. Crack the 2 eggs into the pan and cook until the whites are set and the yolks are still runny.
3. Toast the 2 slices of whole grain bread in a toaster or toaster oven.
4. Plate the eggs and toast, then top with the fresh fruit.

Nutrition Information (per serving):
Calories: 294

Fat: 10 g

Carbohydrates: 31 g

Protein: 16 g

Snack: 1 cup of plain Greek yoghurt, ½ cup of almonds.

Ingredients:

- yoghurt and Almonds
- 1 cup of plain Greek yoghurt
- ½ cup of almonds

Instructions:

1. Place the plain Greek yoghurt in a bowl.
2. Top with ½ cup of almonds.

Nutrition Information (per serving):

Calories: 353

Fat: 20 g

Carbohydrates: 17 g

Protein: 25 g

Lunch: Grilled Chicken Quinoa and Vegetables

Ingredients:

- 4-ounce grilled chicken breast
- ½ cup of cooked quinoa
- 1 cup of steamed vegetables

Instructions:

1. Heat a non-stick skillet over medium-high heat.
2. Place the 4-ounce chicken breast in the skillet and cook for 4-5 minutes per side until cooked through.

3. Heat the cooked quinoa and steamed vegetables in a microwave-safe dish for 1-2 minutes.

4. Plate the chicken, quinoa, and vegetables.

Nutrition Information (per serving):
Calories: 330
Fat: 7 g
Carbohydrates: 31 g
Protein: 36 g

Snack: Egg Toast

Ingredients:
- hard-boiled egg
- slices of whole wheat toast

Instructions:
1. Boil a pot of water and add the egg.
2. Let the egg boil for 8-10 minutes.
3. Toast the 2 slices of whole wheat bread in a toaster or toaster oven.
4. Plate the hard-boiled egg and toast.

Nutrition Information (per serving):
Calories: 230
Fat: 8 g
Carbohydrates: 25 g
Protein: 12 g

Dinner: Salmon Cauliflower and Rice

Ingredients:
- 4-ounce salmon fillet
- 1 cup of roasted cauliflower
- ½ cup of cooked brown rice

Instructions:

1. Preheat the oven to 400° F.

2. Place the 4-ounce salmon fillet on a baking sheet lined with parchment paper.

3. Roast the salmon for 10-12 minutes, or until cooked through.

4. Heat the cooked brown rice and roasted cauliflower in a microwave-safe dish for 1-2 minutes.

5. Plate the salmon, rice, and cauliflower.

Nutrition Information (per serving):
Calories: 375
Fat: 13 g
Carbohydrates: 32 g
Protein: 30 g

DAY 2
Breakfast: Oatmeal with Blueberries and Walnuts

Ingredients:
- 1 cup of rolled oats
- 1 cup of skim milk
- 2 tablespoons of chopped walnuts
- 2 tablespoons of fresh blueberries

Instructions:

1.In a medium pot, bring the milk to a boil.

2.Stir in the oats and walnuts and reduce the heat to low.

3.Simmer for 3-5 minutes, stirring occasionally.

4.Remove from heat and stir in the blueberries.

5.Serve warm.

Nutrition Information (per serving):

Calories: 260

Fat: 7g

Carbohydrates: 36g

Protein: 11g

Snack: Apple and Cottage Cheese

Ingredients:

- 1 apple
- ½ cup of low-fat cottage cheese

Instructions:

1.Wash and slice the apple.

2. Serve with the cottage cheese.

Nutrition Information (per serving):

Calories: 110

Fat: 1g

Carbohydrates: 17g

Protein: 9g

Lunch: Turkey Wrap

Ingredients:
- 2 (8-inch) whole wheat tortillas
- 4 ounces of sliced turkey
- 1 cup of shredded lettuce
- 1 tomato, diced
- 1 avocado, sliced
- 1 cup of fresh fruit

Instructions:
1.Lay the tortillas flat and spread the turkey on top.
2. Top with lettuce, tomato, and avocado.
3. Roll up the tortillas and cut into halves.
4. Serve with the fresh fruit.

Nutrition Information (per serving):
Calories: 390
Fat: 19g
Carbohydrates: 35g
Protein: 23g

Snack: Greek yoghurt and Almonds

Ingredients:
- 1 cup of plain Greek yoghurt
- ½ cup of almonds

Instructions:
1.Mix the yoghurt and almonds together.
2. Serve chilled.

Nutrition Information (per serving):
Calories: 370
Fat: 21g
Carbohydrates: 19g
Protein: 24g

Dinner: Grilled Chicken and Quinoa Bowl

Ingredients:
- 4 ounces of grilled chicken breast
- ½ cup of cooked quinoa
- 1 cup of steamed vegetables

Instructions:
1.Place the chicken, quinoa, and vegetables into a bowl.
2. Mix together and serve.

Nutrition Information (per serving):
Calories: 400
Fat: 8g
Carbohydrates: 35g
Protein: 42g

DAY 3
Breakfast: Egg White Omelet with Spinach, Mushrooms, and Tomatoes

Ingredients:
- 4 egg whites
- ½ cup spinach
- ½ cup mushrooms, diced
- ½ cup tomatoes, diced

- Salt and pepper, to taste

Instructions:

1. Heat a non-stick skillet over medium heat.
2. Add the egg whites and scramble for about 2 minutes.
3. Add the spinach, mushrooms, and tomatoes, and cook for another 3 minutes.
4. Sprinkle with salt and pepper, to taste.
5. Serve with 2 slices of whole grain toast.

Nutrition Information (per serving):
Calories: 152
Fat: 2.7g
Carbohydrates: 12.9g
Protein: 17g

Snack: 1 Cup Plain Greek yoghurt, ½ Cup Almonds

Ingredients:

- 1 cup plain Greek yoghurt
- ½ cup almonds, chopped

Instructions:

1. Place the Greek yoghurt into a bowl.
2. Top with chopped almonds.
3. Serve.

Nutrition Information (per serving):
Calories: 334
Fat: 20.7g
Carbohydrates: 15.8g
Protein: 19.2g

Lunch: Bean and Vegetable Soup

Ingredients:
- 1 can black beans, drained and rinsed
- 1 can cannellini beans, drained and rinsed
- 1 onion, diced
- 1 bell pepper, diced
- 2 cloves garlic, minced
- 1 teaspoon smoked paprika
- 1 teaspoon cumin
- 2 cups vegetable broth
- 2 cups water
- 1 cup cherry tomatoes, halved
- 2 tablespoons fresh parsley, chopped
- Salt and pepper, to taste

Instructions:
1. Heat a large pot over medium-high heat.
2. Add the onion, bell pepper, and garlic, and cook until softened, about 5 minutes.
3. Add the smoked paprika and cumin and cook for another minute.
4. Add the beans, vegetable broth, and water. Bring to a boil.
5. Reduce heat to medium-low and simmer for 20 minutes.
6. Add the tomatoes and parsley and simmer for another 10 minutes.
7. Season with salt and pepper, to taste.
8. Serve with 1 slice of whole wheat bread.

Nutrition Information (per serving):
Calories: 266
Fat: 2.2g

Carbohydrates: 46.3g
Protein: 13.3g

Snack: 1 Hard-Boiled Egg, 2 Slices of Whole Wheat Toast

Ingredients:
- 1 large egg, hard-boiled
- 2 slices of whole wheat toast

Instructions:
1. Hard-boil the egg.
2. Toast the slices of whole wheat bread.
3. Serve the egg and toast.

Nutrition Information (per serving):
Calories: 197
Fat: 6.3g
Carbohydrates: 23.2g
Protein: 13.3g

Dinner: 4-Ounce Grilled Salmon Fillet, 1 Cup Roasted Cauliflower, ½ Cup Cooked Brown Rice

Ingredients:
- 4-ounce salmon fillet
- 1 cup cauliflower, chopped
- 2 tablespoons olive oil
- Salt and pepper, to taste
- ½ cup cooked brown rice

Instructions:
1. Preheat the oven to 400°F.2. Place the cauliflower on a baking sheet and drizzle with olive oil. Sprinkle with salt and pepper, to taste.
3. Roast for 20 minutes.
4. Meanwhile, heat a greased grill pan over medium-high heat.
5. Add the salmon fillet and cook for 3-4 minutes per side.
6. Serve the salmon fillet, roasted cauliflower, and cooked brown rice.

Nutrition Information (per serving):
Calories: 442
Fat: 19.2g
Carbohydrates: 34.1g
Protein: 32.3g

DAY 4
Breakfast: Overnight Oats with Banana and Walnuts

Ingredients:
- 1 cup oats
- 1 banana, sliced
- ¼ cup walnuts
- 1 cup skim milk

Instructions:
1. In a bowl, combine oats, banana slices, and walnuts.
2. Pour in the skim milk and stir to combine.
3. Cover and refrigerate overnight.
4. In the morning, stir the mixture and enjoy.

Nutrition Information (per serving):
Calories: 400
Carbohydrates: 43g
Protein: 13g
Fat: 18g

Snack: Apple and Low-Fat Cottage Cheese

Ingredients:
- 1 apple, sliced
- ½ cup low-fat cottage cheese

Instructions:
1. Slice the apple and divide into small pieces.
2. Place the apple slices in a bowl and top with cottage cheese.
3. Enjoy!

Nutrition Information (per serving):
Calories: 145
Carbohydrates: 18g
Protein: 12g
Fat: 4g

Lunch: Spinach Salad with Grilled Chicken

Ingredients:
- 2 cups fresh spinach
- 4 ounces grilled chicken, diced
- 1 cup fresh fruit, diced
- 2 tablespoons extra-virgin olive oil
- 2 tablespoons balsamic vinegar

Instructions:

1. In a large bowl, combine spinach, chicken, and fruit.
2. Drizzle with oil and vinegar and toss to combine.
3. Enjoy!

Nutrition Information (per serving):
Calories: 350
Carbohydrates: 20g
Protein: 28g
Fat: 17g

Snack: **Greek yoghurt and Almonds**

Ingredients:
- 1 cup plain Greek yoghurt
- ½ cup almonds

Instructions:

1. Scoop the Greek yoghurt into a bowl.
2. Top with almonds and enjoy.

Nutrition Information (per serving):
Calories: 495
Carbohydrates: 20g
Protein: 25g
Fat: 35g

Dinner: **Grilled Chicken Breast with Quinoa and Steamed Vegetables**

Ingredients:
- 4 ounces grilled chicken breast

- ½ cup cooked quinoa
- 1 cup steamed vegetables of your choice
- 1 tablespoon extra-virgin olive oil

Instructions:

1. Place the chicken breast and quinoa in a large bowl.

2. Add the steamed vegetables and drizzle with oil.

3. Toss to combine and enjoy.

Nutrition Information (per serving):

Calories: 365

Carbohydrates: 20g

Protein: 37g

Fat: 12g

DAY 5

Breakfast: **Smoothie**

Ingredients:

- 1 banana
- 1 cup of almond milk
- 1 scoop of protein powder

Instructions:

1. Peel and slice banana into chunks.

2. Place banana, almond milk, and protein powder into blender and blend until smooth.

3. Pour into a glass and enjoy!

Nutrition Information (per serving):

Calories: 200

Fat: 4g

Protein: 14g

Carbohydrates: 26g

Snack: Greek yoghurt and Almonds

Ingredients:
- 1 cup of plain Greek yoghurt
- ½ cup of almonds

Instructions:
1. Place Greek yoghurt and almonds in a bowl and stir until combined.
2. Enjoy!

Nutrition Information (per serving):
Calories: 360
Fat: 18g
Protein: 28g
Carbohydrates: 18g

Lunch: Hummus Wrap

Ingredients:
- 1 whole wheat tortilla
- 2 tablespoons of hummus
- 1 lettuce leaf
- 2 slices of tomato
- 2 slices of cucumber
- 1 cup of fresh fruit

Instructions:
1. Spread hummus onto tortilla.
2. Place lettuce, tomato, and cucumber onto tortilla.
3. Roll up tortilla and enjoy with fresh fruit.

Nutrition Information (per serving):
Calories: 340
Fat: 10g
Protein: 11g
Carbohydrates: 50g

Snack: Hard Boiled Egg and Toast

Ingredients:
- 1 hard-boiled egg
- 2 slices of whole wheat toast

Instructions:
1. Peel and slice hard-boiled egg.
2. Toast bread and spread egg slices on top.
3. Enjoy!

Nutrition Information (per serving):
Calories: 280
Fat: 8g
Protein: 16g
Carbohydrates: 34g

Dinner: Grilled Salmon and Cauliflower Rice

Ingredients:
- 4-ounce grilled salmon fillet
- 1 cup of roasted cauliflower
- ½ cup of cooked brown rice

Instructions:
1. Preheat oven to 375°F.

2. Place salmon on baking sheet and roast for 15 minutes.

3. Place cauliflower and rice into a bowl and mix together.

4. Place salmon and cauliflower rice onto plate and enjoy!

Nutrition Information (per serving):
Calories: 390
Fat: 16g
Protein: 33g
Carbohydrates: 27g

DAY 6
Breakfast: 2 Eggs Over-Easy

Ingredients:
- 2 eggs
- 2 slices of whole grain toast
- ½ cup of fresh fruit

Instructions:
1. Heat a non-stick pan over medium heat.
2. Crack eggs into the pan and cook until the whites are set and the yolks are still runny.
3. Toast the whole grain toast.
4. Serve eggs over toast with fresh fruit.

Nutrition Information (per serving):
Calories: 277
Fat: 11g
Carbohydrates: 27g
Protein: 16g

Snack: 1 Apple, ½ Cup of Low-Fat Cottage Cheese

Ingredients:
- 1 apple
- ½ cup of low-fat cottage cheese

Instructions:
1. Slice the apple and serve with cottage cheese.

Nutrition Information (per serving):
Calories: 158
Fat: 2.5g
Carbohydrates: 25g
Protein: 11g

Lunch: Grilled Vegetable Wrap with Hummus

Ingredients:
- 1 whole wheat wrap
- 2 tablespoons of hummus
- ½ cup of grilled vegetables (such as bell peppers, zucchini, and mushrooms)
- 1 cup of fresh fruit

Instructions:
1. Preheat grill or grill pan over medium heat.
2. Grill vegetables until lightly charred and tender.
3. Spread hummus on the wrap.
4. Add grilled vegetables.
5. Roll up wrap and cut in half.
6. Serve with fresh fruit.

Nutrition Information (per serving):
Calories: 295
Fat: 5g
Carbohydrates: 46g
Protein: 10g

Snack: 1 Cup of Plain Greek yoghurt, ½ Cup of Almonds

Ingredients:
- 1 cup of plain Greek yoghurt
- ½ cup of almonds

Instructions:
1. Place Greek yoghurt in a bowl.
2. Top with almonds.

Nutrition Information (per serving):
Calories: 308
Fat: 18g
Carbohydrates: 16g
Protein: 17g

Dinner: 4-Ounce Grilled Chicken Breast, ½ Cup of Cooked Quinoa, 1 Cup of Steamed Vegetables

Ingredients:
- 4-ounce grilled chicken breast
- ½ cup of cooked quinoa
- 1 cup of steamed vegetables (such as broccoli, carrots, and peas)

Instructions:
1. Preheat grill or grill pan over medium heat.

2. Grill chicken until cooked through, about 5 minutes per side.
3. Cook quinoa according to package Instructions: .
4. Steam vegetables until tender.
5. Serve chicken with quinoa and vegetables.

Nutrition Information (per serving):
Calories: 317
Fat: 7g
Carbohydrates: 22g
Protein: 34g

DAY 7
Breakfast: Oatmeal with Blueberries and Walnuts

Ingredients:
- 1 cup of rolled oats
- 1 cup of skim milk
- 1/4 cup of blueberries
- 2 tablespoons of chopped walnuts

Instructions:
1. In a medium saucepan, bring the milk to a boil.
2. Add the oats and reduce the heat to medium-low. Simmer for 5 minutes, stirring occasionally.
3. Remove from heat and stir in the blueberries and walnuts.
4. Serve warm.

Nutrition Information (per serving):
Calories: 341
Fat: 8.2g
Carbohydrates: 53.7g

Protein: 11.9g.

Snack: Hard-Boiled Egg and Toast

Ingredients:
- 1 hard-boiled egg
- 2 slices of whole wheat toast

Instructions:
1. Bring a small pot of water to a boil.
2. Carefully add the egg and boil for 10 minutes.
3. Remove from heat and run cold water over the egg until it is cool enough to handle.
4. Peel the egg and cut in half.
5. Toast the bread and serve with the egg.

Nutrition Information (per serving):
Calories: 234
Fat: 9.8g
Carbohydrates: 25.2g
Protein: 11.7g.

Lunch: Tuna Salad Sandwich

Ingredients:
- 1 can of tuna, drained
- 2 tablespoons of light mayonnaise
- 2 slices of whole wheat bread
- 1 cup of fresh fruit

Instructions:
1. In a medium bowl, combine the tuna and mayonnaise.
2. Spread the tuna mixture on one slice of bread.

3. Top with the other slice of bread.
4. Serve with the fresh fruit.

Nutrition Information (per serving):
Calories: 442
Fat: 11.3g
Carbohydrates: 58.1g
Protein: 28.2g.

Snack: Greek yoghurt and Almonds

Ingredients:
- 1 cup of plain Greek yoghurt
- ½ cup of almonds

Instructions:
1. Place the yoghurt in a bowl.
2. Top with the almonds.
3. Serve.

Nutrition Information (per serving):
Calories: 449
Fat: 25.3g
Carbohydrates: 28.9g
Protein: 24.6g.

Dinner: Grilled Salmon and Roasted Cauliflower

Ingredients:
- 4-ounce grilled salmon fillet
- 1 cup of roasted cauliflower
- ½ cup of cooked brown rice

Instructions:
1. Preheat oven to 400°F.
2. Place the cauliflower on a baking sheet and roast for 15 minutes.
3. Remove from oven and set aside.
4. Heat a grill or grill pan to medium-high heat.
5. Grill the salmon for 4-5 minutes per side.
6. Serve the salmon with the roasted cauliflower and cooked brown rice.

Nutrition Information (per serving):
Calories: 486
Fat: 17.8g
Carbohydrates: 48.1g
Protein: 32.3g.

WEEK 2

Day 8:
Breakfast: Egg white omelette with spinach, mushrooms, and tomatoes, 2 slices of whole grain toast.
Snack: 1 apple, ½ cup of low-fat cottage cheese.
Lunch: Turkey and vegetable wrap with hummus, 1 cup of fresh fruit.
Snack: 1 cup of plain Greek yoghurt, ½ cup of almonds.
Dinner: 4-ounce grilled chicken breast, ½ cup of cooked quinoa, 1 cup of steamed vegetables.

Day 9:

Breakfast: Smoothie with banana, almond milk, and protein powder.

Snack: 1 hard-boiled egg, 2 slices of whole wheat toast.

Lunch: Bean and vegetable soup, 1 slice of whole wheat bread.

Snack: 1 cup of plain Greek yoghurt, ½ cup of almonds.

Dinner: 4-ounce grilled salmon fillet, 1 cup of roasted cauliflower, ½ cup of cooked brown rice.

Day 10:

Breakfast: Overnight oats with banana and walnuts, 1 cup of skim milk.

Snack: 1 apple, ½ cup of low-fat cottage cheese.

Lunch: Spinach salad with grilled chicken, 1 cup of fresh fruit.

Snack: 1 cup of plain Greek yoghurt, ½ cup of almonds.

Dinner: 4-ounce grilled chicken breast, ½ cup of cooked quinoa, 1 cup of steamed vegetables.

Day 11:

Breakfast: 2 eggs over-easy, 2 slices of whole grain toast, ½ cup of fresh fruit.

Snack: 1 hard-boiled egg, 2 slices of whole wheat toast.

Lunch: Hummus wrap with lettuce, tomato, and cucumber, 1 cup of fresh fruit.

Snack: 1 cup of plain Greek yoghurt, ½ cup of almonds.

Dinner: 4-ounce grilled salmon fillet, 1 cup of roasted cauliflower, ½ cup of cooked brown rice.

Day 12:

Breakfast: Oatmeal with blueberries and walnuts, 1 cup of skim milk.

Snack: 1 apple, ½ cup of low-fat cottage cheese.

Lunch: Tuna salad sandwich on whole wheat bread, 1 cup of fresh fruit.

Snack: 1 cup of plain Greek yoghurt, ½ cup of almonds.

Dinner: 4-ounce grilled chicken breast, ½ cup of cooked quinoa, 1 cup of steamed vegetables.

Day 13:

Breakfast: Egg white omelet with spinach, mushrooms, and tomatoes, 2 slices of whole grain toast.

Snack: 1 hard-boiled egg, 2 slices of whole wheat toast.

Lunch: Grilled vegetable wrap with hummus, 1 cup of fresh fruit.

Snack: 1 cup of plain Greek yoghurt, ½ cup of almonds.

Dinner: 4-ounce grilled salmon fillet, 1 cup of roasted cauliflower, ½ cup of cooked brown rice.

Day 14:

Breakfast: Smoothie with banana, almond milk, and protein powder.

Snack: 1 apple, ½ cup of low-fat cottage cheese.

Lunch: Turkey wrap with lettuce, tomato, and avocado, 1 cup of fresh fruit.

Snack: 1 cup of plain Greek yoghurt, ½ cup of almonds.

Dinner: 4-ounce grilled chicken breast, ½ cup of cooked quinoa, 1 cup of steamed vegetables.

Grocery Shopping List for WEEK 2

Protein:
- 28 eggs (14 for 2 omelettes, 2 for each snack)
- 16 ounces of grilled chicken breast (8 ounces for each dinner)
- 8 ounces of salmon fillet
- 8 ounces of turkey breast (for lunch day 8)
- 1 can of tuna (for lunch day 12)

Dairy/Dairy Alternatives:
- 4 cups of plain Greek yoghurt (for snacks and lunch)
- 2 cups of low-fat cottage cheese (for snacks)
- 4 cups of skim milk (for breakfasts and snacks)
- Almond milk (for smoothies)

Fruits:
- Fresh fruit (choose a variety of your favorites such as blueberries, bananas, apples)
- 2 cups of blueberries
- 7 apples (1 for each snack)
- 7 cups of fresh fruit (1 cup for each lunch)

Vegetables:
- 7 cups of spinach (1 cup for each lunch)
- 6 cups of roasted cauliflower (1 cup for each dinner)
- 10 cups of steamed vegetables (1 cup for each lunch and dinner)
- 7 cups of grilled veggies (for lunch day 6)

Grains/Breads:
- 40 slices of whole grain toast (4 per breakfast)
- 10 wraps/tortillas (for lunch and dinner)
- 2 cups of cooked quinoa (1/2 cup for each dinner)
- 1 loaf of whole wheat bread (for lunch day 3 and day 14)
- 1 cup of cooked brown rice (for dinner day 1 and day 14)
- Oats (for overnight oats)

Nuts/Seeds:
- 3 cups of almonds (1/2 cup for each snack and 1/2 cup for a snack on day 2)
- Walnuts (for breakfast day 2 and day 12)

Miscellaneous:
- Bean and vegetable soup (can or ingredients to make homemade)
- Hummus (for lunch and dinner)
- Lettuce (for lunch and dinner wraps)
- Tomato (for wraps and salads)
- Avocado (for lunch day 2)
- Cucumber (for wraps and salads)
- Protein powder (for smoothies)
- Seasonings and spices as desired

DAY 8

Breakfast: Egg White Omelet with Spinach, Mushrooms, and Tomatoes

Ingredients:
- 3 egg whites
- ¼ cup of spinach, chopped
- ¼ cup of mushrooms, chopped
- ¼ cup of tomatoes, chopped
- 2 slices of whole grain toast

Instructions:
1. Heat a nonstick pan over medium heat.
2. Add the egg whites and cook for about 1 minute, stirring occasionally.
3. Add the spinach, mushrooms, and tomatoes, and cook for another few minutes until the egg whites are cooked through.
4. Serve with two slices of whole grain toast.

Nutrition Information (per serving):
Calories: 224
Protein: 14g
Fat: 4g
Carbohydrates: 29g

Snack: 1 Apple, ½ Cup of Low-Fat Cottage Cheese

Ingredients:
- 1 apple
- ½ cup of low-fat cottage cheese

Instructions:
1. Slice the apple into wedges or cubes.
2. Place the apple slices and cottage cheese in a bowl and mix together.

Nutrition Information (per serving):
Calories: 126
Protein: 11g
Fat: 1g
Carbohydrates: 20g

Lunch: Turkey and Vegetable Wrap with Hummus

Ingredients:
- 1 whole wheat wrap
- 3 ounces of sliced turkey
- ¼ cup of shredded carrots
- ¼ cup of spinach, chopped
- ¼ cup of cucumber, chopped
- 2 tablespoons of hummus

Instructions:
1. Place the wrap flat on a plate or cutting board.
2. Arrange the turkey, carrots, spinach, and cucumber in a line down the center of the wrap.
3. Spread the hummus over the vegetables.
4. Fold the edges of the wrap over the filling, and then roll it up tightly.

Nutrition Information (per serving):
Calories: 263
Protein: 19g

Fat: 6g

Carbohydrates: 34g

Snack: 1 Cup of Plain Greek yoghurt, ½ Cup of Almonds

Ingredients:

- 1 cup of plain Greek yoghurt
- ½ cup of almonds

Instructions:

1. Place the yoghurt in a bowl.
2. Top with almonds.

Nutrition Information (per serving):

Calories: 403

Protein: 23g

Fat: 24g

Carbohydrates: 21g

Dinner: 4-Ounce Grilled Chicken Breast, ½ Cup of Cooked Quinoa, 1 Cup of Steamed Vegetables

Ingredients:

- 4-ounce grilled chicken breast
- ½ cup of cooked quinoa
- 1 cup of steamed vegetables (such as broccoli, cauliflower, carrots, etc.)

Instructions:

1. Preheat the oven to 350°F.
2. Place the chicken breast in an oven-safe dish and bake for 20 minutes, or until cooked through.
3. Meanwhile, cook the quinoa according to package instructions.

4. Steam the vegetables in a steamer basket over boiling water until tender.

5. Serve the chicken, quinoa, and vegetables together.

Nutrition Information (per serving):

Calories: 283

Protein: 33g

Fat: 5g

Carbohydrates: 25g

DAY 9

Breakfast: Banana Almond Protein Smoothie

Ingredients:

- 1 banana
- 1 cup almond milk
- 1 scoop protein powder

Instructions:

1. Place banana, almond milk, and protein powder in a blender.

2. Blend until smooth.

3. Pour into a glass and enjoy!

Nutrition Information (per serving):

Calories: 224

Fat: 4.5g

Carbohydrates: 24.8g

Protein: 20.3g

Snack: Hard-Boiled Egg and Toast

Ingredients:
- 1 hard-boiled egg
- 2 slices of whole wheat toast

Instructions:
1. Boil one egg for 8 minutes.
2. Toast two slices of whole wheat toast.
3. Slice the egg and place on top of the toast.

Nutrition Information (per serving):
Calories: 207
Fat: 7.4g
Carbohydrates: 24.1g
Protein: 11.2g

Lunch: Bean and Vegetable Soup

Ingredients:
- 1 can of white beans
- 1 cup of diced carrots
- 1 cup of diced celery
- 1 cup of diced onion
- 3 cups of vegetable broth

Instructions:
1. Place all ingredients in a large pot and bring to a boil.
2. Reduce heat and simmer for 20 minutes, stirring occasionally.
3. Serve with a slice of whole wheat bread.

Nutrition Information (per serving):
Calories: 133
Fat: 0.3g
Carbohydrates: 24.8g
Protein: 8.1g

Snack: Plain Greek yoghurt with Almonds

Ingredients:
- 1 cup of plain Greek yoghurt
- ½ cup of almonds

Instructions:
1. Place yoghurt in a bowl.
2. Top with almonds.
3. Enjoy!

Nutrition Information (per serving):
Calories: 476
Fat: 28.0g
Carbohydrates: 24.5g
Protein: 27.4g

Dinner: Grilled Salmon with Roasted Cauliflower and Brown Rice

Ingredients:
- 4-ounce grilled salmon fillet
- 1 cup of roasted cauliflower
- ½ cup of cooked brown rice

Instructions:
1. Preheat oven to 425°F.

2. Place the salmon fillet on a greased baking sheet and cook for 12-15 minutes, or until cooked through.
3. Meanwhile, roast cauliflower on a greased baking sheet for 20 minutes.
4. Cook brown rice according to package instructions.
5. Serve salmon with roasted cauliflower and brown rice.

Nutrition Information (per serving):
Calories: 461
Fat: 17.7g
Carbohydrates: 40.5g
Protein: 28.9g

DAY 10
Breakfast: Overnight Oats with Banana and Walnuts

Ingredients:
- 1/2 cup rolled oats
- 1/2 cup skim milk
- 1/2 banana, mashed
- 1 tablespoon honey
- 1/4 teaspoon ground cinnamon
- 1 tablespoon chopped walnuts

Instructions:
1. In a medium bowl, combine the oats and milk. Stir in the mashed banana, honey, and cinnamon.
2. Cover the bowl and refrigerate overnight.
3. In the morning, stir in the chopped walnuts.
4. Serve with additional milk, if desired.

Nutrition Information (per serving):
Calories: 211
Fat: 4.8g
Carbohydrate: 34.3g
Protein: 7.8g

Snack: Apple and Low-fat Cottage Cheese

Ingredients:
- 1 apple
- 1/2 cup low-fat cottage cheese

Instructions:
1. Slice the apple and serve with the cottage cheese.

Nutrition Information (per serving):
Calories: 135
Fat: 1.3g
Carbohydrate: 22.3g
Protein: 10.2g

Lunch: Spinach Salad with Grilled Chicken

Ingredients:
- 2 cups of fresh spinach
- 1/4 cup of cherry tomatoes, halved
- 1/4 cup of red onion, diced
- 2 ounces of grilled chicken
- 1 cup of fresh fruit (optional)

Instructions:
1. In a large bowl, combine the spinach, tomatoes, and onion.
2. Top with the grilled chicken and fruit.

Nutrition Information (per serving):
Calories: 183
Fat: 3.1g
Carbohydrate: 15.2g
Protein: 24.5g

Snack: Plain Greek yoghurt with Almonds

Ingredients:
- 1 cup of plain Greek yoghurt
- 1/2 cup of almonds

Instructions:
1. In a bowl, combine the Greek yoghurt and almonds.
2. Serve.

Nutrition Information (per serving):
Calories: 431
Fat: 25.7g
Carbohydrate: 22.6g
Protein: 25.6g

Dinner: Grilled Chicken Breast with Quinoa and Steamed Vegetables

Ingredients:
- 4 ounces of grilled chicken breast
- 1/2 cup cooked quinoa
- 1 cup of steamed vegetables (such as broccoli, carrots, and/or bell peppers)

Instructions:
1. Grill the chicken breast.
2. Cook the quinoa according to package instructions.
3. Steam the vegetables.
4. Serve the chicken, quinoa, and vegetables together.

Nutrition Information (per serving):
Calories: 288
Fat: 6.2g
Carbohydrate: 28.0g
Protein: 29.7g

DAY 11
Breakfast: 2 Eggs Over-Easy with Toast and Fresh Fruit

Ingredients:
- 2 eggs
- 2 slices of whole grain bread
- ½ cup of fresh fruit

Instructions:
1. Heat a large non-stick skillet over medium-high heat.
2. Crack the eggs into the pan and season with salt and pepper.
3. Cook the eggs for 2 to 3 minutes, or until the whites are cooked through and the yolks are still runny.
4. Remove the eggs from the heat and transfer to a plate.
5. Toast the bread in a toaster until golden brown.
6. Serve the eggs and toast with the fresh fruit.

Nutrition Information (per serving):

Calories: 357

Fat: 14 g

Carbohydrates: 32 g

Protein: 19 g

Snack: Hard-Boiled Egg and Toast

Ingredients:
- 1 hard-boiled egg
- 2 slices of whole wheat toast

Instructions:

1. Place the egg in a pot of cold water and bring to a boil.

2. Once boiling, reduce the heat to low and simmer for 10 minutes.

3. Remove the egg from the pot and let cool.

4. Toast the bread in a toaster until golden brown.

5. Peel and slice the egg and serve with the toast.

Nutrition Information (per serving):

Calories: 166

Fat: 7 g

Carbohydrates: 14 g

Protein: 11 g

Lunch: Hummus Wrap with Lettuce, Tomato, and Cucumber

Ingredients:
- 1 whole wheat wrap
- 2 tablespoons of hummus
- Lettuce, tomato, and cucumber slices

- 1 cup of fresh fruit

Instructions:

1. Spread the hummus on the wrap.
2. Arrange the lettuce, tomato, and cucumber slices on top of the hummus.
3. Roll up the wrap and cut in half.
4. Serve with the fresh fruit.

Nutrition Information (per serving):
Calories: 270
Fat: 6 g
Carbohydrates: 42 g
Protein: 10 g

Snack: Greek yoghurt and Almonds

Ingredients:

- 1 cup of plain Greek yoghurt
- ½ cup of almonds

Instructions:

1. Place the yoghurt in a bowl.
2. Top with the almonds.
3. Enjoy!

Nutrition Information (per serving):
Calories: 326
Fat: 14 g
Carbohydrates: 19 g
Protein: 24 g

Dinner: Grilled Salmon Fillet with Roasted Cauliflower and Brown Rice

Ingredients:
- 4-ounce grilled salmon fillet
- 1 cup of roasted cauliflower
- ½ cup of cooked brown rice

Instructions:

1. Preheat the oven to 425°F.

2. Place the salmon fillet on a baking sheet lined with parchment paper and season with salt and pepper.

3. Bake for 8 to 10 minutes, or until cooked through.

4. Place the cauliflower on a baking sheet lined with parchment paper and season with salt and pepper.

5. Roast for 15 minutes, or until lightly golden and tender.

6. Serve the salmon with the roasted cauliflower and brown rice.

Nutrition Information (per serving):
Calories: 441
Fat: 18 g
Carbohydrates: 32 g
Protein: 36 g

DAY 12

Breakfast: Oatmeal with Blueberries and Walnuts

Ingredients:
- 1 cup rolled oats
- 1 cup skim milk
- ¼ cup walnuts

- ¼ cup fresh or frozen blueberries

Instructions:

1. In a medium pot, bring the milk to a simmer over medium heat.

2. Add the oats and cook for about 5 minutes, stirring occasionally.

3. Remove from heat and stir in the walnuts and blueberries.

4. Serve warm.

Nutrition Information (per serving):

Calories: 405

Fat: 13 g

Carbohydrates: 51 g

Protein: 18 g

Snack: Apple with Low-Fat Cottage Cheese

Ingredients:
- 1 medium apple
- ½ cup low-fat cottage cheese

Instructions:

1. Slice the apple and arrange on a plate.

2. Top with cottage cheese.

3. Enjoy.

Nutrition Information (per serving):

Calories: 140

Fat: 2 g

Carbohydrates: 21 g

Protein: 14 g

Lunch: Tuna Salad Sandwich on Whole Wheat Bread

Ingredients:
- 2 slices of whole wheat bread
- 3 ounces of canned tuna
- 3 tablespoons light mayonnaise
- 1 teaspoon Dijon mustard
- 1 cup fresh fruit

Instructions:
1. In a small bowl, combine the tuna, mayonnaise, and mustard.
2. Spread the tuna salad onto the two slices of whole wheat bread.
3. Serve with fresh fruit.

Nutrition Information (per serving):
Calories: 369
Fat: 10 g
Carbohydrates: 46 g
Protein: 24 g

Snack: Plain Greek yoghurt with Almonds

Ingredients:
- 1 cup plain Greek yoghurt
- ½ cup almonds

Instructions:
1. In a bowl, combine the Greek yoghurt and almonds.
2. Enjoy.

Nutrition Information (per serving):
Calories: 416
Fat: 24 g
Carbohydrates: 18 g
Protein: 28 g

Dinner: Grilled Chicken Breast with Quinoa and Steamed Vegetables

Ingredients:
- 4 ounces grilled chicken breast
- ½ cup cooked quinoa
- 1 cup steamed vegetables

Instructions:
1. Grill the chicken breast until cooked through.
2. In a bowl, combine the cooked quinoa and steamed vegetables.
3. Serve the chicken with the quinoa and vegetables.

Nutrition Information (per serving):
Calories: 341
Fat: 8 g
Carbohydrates: 30 g
Protein: 33 g

DAY 13
Breakfast: Egg White Omelet with Spinach, Mushrooms, and Tomatoes

Ingredients:
- 4 egg whites

- 1/4 cup chopped spinach
- 1/4 cup chopped mushrooms
- 1/4 cup chopped tomatoes
- 2 slices of whole grain toast

Instructions:

1. Heat a large non-stick skillet over medium heat.

2. Add the egg whites to the skillet and cook for 2-3 minutes, stirring occasionally, until the egg whites are cooked through and no longer runny.

3. Add the spinach, mushrooms, and tomatoes to the skillet and cook for an additional 2-3 minutes.

4. To assemble the omelet, fold the egg whites over the vegetables and cook until the omelet is golden brown.

5. Serve with the slices of toast.

Nutrition Information (per serving):
Calories: 250
Fat: 4g
Carbohydrates: 31g
Protein: 21g

Snack: Hard-Boiled Egg and Toast

Ingredients:

- 1 hard-boiled egg
- 2 slices of whole wheat toast

Instructions:

1. Peel the hard-boiled egg and cut into slices.

2. Toast the slices of whole wheat toast.

3. Serve the egg slices and toast together.

Nutrition Information (per serving):
Calories: 216
Fat: 7g
Carbohydrates: 26g
Protein: 12g

Lunch: Grilled Vegetable Wrap with Hummus

Ingredients:
- 1 whole wheat wrap
- 2 tablespoons of hummus
- 1/2 cup of chopped grilled vegetables (such as bell peppers, onions, mushrooms, and zucchini)
- 1 cup of fresh fruit

Instructions:
1. Preheat the grill or grill pan over medium heat.
2. Grill the vegetables until lightly charred and cooked through, about 5 minutes.
3. Spread the hummus onto the wrap and top with the grilled vegetables.
4. Roll up the wrap and cut in half.
5. Serve with the fresh fruit.

Nutrition Information (per serving):
Calories: 279
Fat: 5g
Carbohydrates: 48g
Protein: 11g

Snack: Plain Greek yoghurt with Almonds

Ingredients:
- 1 cup of plain Greek yoghurt
- 1/2 cup of almonds

Instructions:
1. Place the yoghurt into a bowl.
2. Top with the almonds.
3. Enjoy!

Nutrition Information (per serving):
Calories: 352
Fat: 22g
Carbohydrates: 18g
Protein: 19g

Dinner: Grilled Salmon Fillet, Roasted Cauliflower, and Brown Rice

Ingredients:
- 4-ounce grilled salmon fillet
- 1 cup of roasted cauliflower
- 1/2 cup of cooked brown rice

Instructions:
1. Preheat the oven to 400 degrees F.
2. Place the salmon fillet on a baking sheet lined with parchment paper.
3. Bake for 10 minutes, or until the salmon is cooked through.
4. Meanwhile, roast the cauliflower in the oven for 15 minutes, stirring halfway through.

5. To assemble the dish, divide the cooked brown rice among plates and top with the grilled salmon and roasted cauliflower.

Nutrition Information (per serving):
Calories: 468
Fat: 15g
Carbohydrates: 45g
Protein: 36g

DAY 14
Breakfast: Smoothie

Ingredients:
- 1 banana
- 2 cups almond milk
- 2 scoops protein powder

Instructions:
1. Place banana, almond milk, and protein powder in a blender.
2. Blend until smooth.
3. Serve and enjoy.

Nutrition Information (per serving):
Calories: 330
Fat: 8g
Carbohydrates: 36g
Protein: 32g

Snack: Apple with Cottage Cheese

Ingredients:
- 1 apple
- 1/2 cup low-fat cottage cheese

Instructions:
1. Slice the apple into wedges.
2. Serve with the cottage cheese.

Nutrition Information (per serving):
Calories: 145
Fat: 2.5g
Carbohydrates: 24g
Protein: 11g

Lunch: Turkey Wrap

Ingredients:
- 2 large tortillas
- 4 ounces turkey breast, thinly sliced
- 1/2 cup lettuce, shredded
- 1/2 tomato, diced
- 1/4 avocado, sliced

Instructions:
1. Lay out the two tortillas.
2. Place the turkey, lettuce, tomato, and avocado on one half of each tortilla.
3. Fold the other half of the tortilla over the filling.
4. Cut in half and serve.

Nutrition Information (per serving):
Calories: 290
Fat: 10g
Carbohydrates: 29g
Protein: 20g

Snack: Greek yoghurt and Almonds

Ingredients:
- 1 cup plain Greek yoghurt
- 1/2 cup almonds

Instructions:
1. Place the Greek yoghurt in a bowl.
2. Top with the almonds.
3. Serve and enjoy.

Nutrition Information (per serving):
Calories: 409
Fat: 26g
Carbohydrates: 18g
Protein: 22g

Dinner: Grilled Chicken, Quinoa, and Vegetables

Ingredients:
- 4 ounces grilled chicken breast
- 1/2 cup cooked quinoa
- 1 cup steamed vegetables

Instructions:
1. Grill the chicken breast until cooked through.
2. Heat the quinoa and vegetables.

3. Serve the grilled chicken, quinoa, and vegetables.

Nutrition Information (per serving):
Calories: 308
Fat: 7g
Carbohydrates: 23g
Protein: 34g

WEEK 3

Day 15:
Breakfast: 2 eggs over-easy, 2 slices of whole grain toast, ½ cup of fresh fruit.
Snack: 1 hard-boiled egg, 2 slices of whole wheat toast.
Lunch: Bean and vegetable soup, 1 slice of whole wheat bread.
Snack: 1 cup of plain Greek yoghurt, ½ cup of almonds.
Dinner: 4-ounce grilled salmon fillet, 1 cup of roasted cauliflower, ½ cup of cooked brown rice.

Day 16:
Breakfast: Overnight oats with banana and walnuts, 1 cup of skim milk.
Snack: 1 apple, ½ cup of low-fat cottage cheese.
Lunch: Spinach salad with grilled chicken, 1 cup of fresh fruit.
Snack: 1 cup of plain Greek yoghurt, ½ cup of almonds.
Dinner: 4-ounce grilled chicken breast, ½ cup of cooked quinoa, 1 cup of steamed vegetables.

Day 17:
Breakfast: Smoothie with banana, almond milk, and protein powder.
Snack: 1 hard-boiled egg, 2 slices of whole wheat toast.
Lunch: Hummus wrap with lettuce, tomato, and cucumber, 1 cup of fresh fruit.
Snack: 1 cup of plain Greek yoghurt, ½ cup of almonds.
Dinner: 4-ounce grilled salmon fillet, 1 cup of roasted cauliflower, ½ cup of cooked brown rice.

Day 18:
Breakfast: Oatmeal with blueberries and walnuts, 1 cup of skim milk.
Snack: 1 apple, ½ cup of low-fat cottage cheese.
Lunch: Turkey and vegetable wrap with hummus, 1 cup of fresh fruit.
Snack: 1 cup of plain Greek yoghurt, ½ cup of almonds.
Dinner: 4-ounce grilled chicken breast, ½ cup of cooked quinoa, 1 cup of steamed vegetables.

Day 19:
Breakfast: Egg white omelet with spinach, mushrooms, and tomatoes, 2 slices of whole grain toast.
Snack: 1 hard-boiled egg, 2 slices of whole wheat toast.
Lunch: Grilled vegetable wrap with hummus, 1 cup of fresh fruit.
Snack: 1 cup of plain Greek yoghurt, ½ cup of almonds.
Dinner: 4-ounce grilled salmon fillet, 1 cup of roasted cauliflower, ½ cup of cooked brown rice.

Day 20:

Breakfast: 2 eggs over-easy, 2 slices of whole grain toast, ½ cup of fresh fruit.

Snack: 1 apple, ½ cup of low-fat cottage cheese.

Lunch: Tuna salad sandwich on whole wheat bread, 1 cup of fresh fruit.

Snack: 1 cup of plain Greek yoghurt, ½ cup of almonds.

Dinner: 4-ounce grilled chicken breast, ½ cup of cooked quinoa, 1 cup of steamed vegetables.

Day 21:

Breakfast: Overnight oats with banana and walnuts, 1 cup of skim milk.

Snack: 1 hard-boiled egg, 2 slices of whole wheat toast.

Lunch: Bean and vegetable soup, 1 slice of whole wheat bread.

Snack: 1 cup of plain Greek yoghurt, ½ cup of almonds.

Dinner: 4-ounce grilled salmon fillet, 1 cup of roasted cauliflower, ½ cup of cooked brown rice.

Grocery Shopping List for WEEK 3

Proteins:
- Eggs: 14
- Salmon fillet: 20 ounces
- Grilled chicken breast: 20 ounces
- Turkey slices: 8 ounces
- Canned tuna: 1 can
- Greek yoghurt: 7 cups
- Low-fat cottage cheese: 2 cups

- Protein powder: 1 container

Grains:
- Whole grain toast: 16 slices
- Whole wheat bread: 8 slices
- Cooked brown rice: 2 cups
- Quinoa: 1 cup
- Oatmeal: 2 cups

Fruits:
- Bananas: 4
- Fresh fruit (of choice): 14 cups
- Blueberries: ½ cup
- Apples: 2

Vegetables:
- Fresh vegetables for soup (of choice): 4 cups
- Roasted cauliflower: 2 cups
- Spinach: 4 cups
- Lettuce: 2 cups
- Tomatoes: 4
- Cucumber: 1
- Mushrooms: 1 cup

Nuts and Seeds:
- Walnuts: ½ cup
- Almonds: 3 cups

Dairy and Refrigerated Items:
- Skim milk: 4 cups
- Hummus: 1 container

Pantry Items:
- Olive oil or cooking spray
- Salt and pepper
- Spices and herbs (to taste)
- Whole wheat wraps: 4

Canned Goods:
- Beans (of choice for soup): 1 can

The amounts mentioned above are estimates and can be adjusted based on personal preferences and portion sizes.

Recipes

DAY 15
Breakfast: Eggs Over-Easy with Toast and Fresh Fruit

Ingredients:
- 2 eggs
- 2 slices of whole grain toast
- ½ cup of fresh fruit

Instructions:
1. Heat a large non-stick skillet over medium heat.
2. Crack two eggs into the skillet and cook for 3-4 minutes until the whites are set and the yolks are still runny.
3. Meanwhile, toast two slices of whole grain bread.
4. Plate the eggs over-easy and toast and top with ½ cup of fresh fruit.

Nutrition Information (per serving):
Calories: 339
Fat: 11 g
Carbohydrates: 38 g
Protein: 20 g

Snack: Hard-Boiled Egg Toast

Ingredients:
- 1 hard-boiled egg
- 2 slices of whole wheat toast

Instructions:
1. Boil one egg.
2. Toast two slices of whole wheat toast.
3. Slice the hard-boiled egg and place on top of the toast.

Nutrition Information (per serving):
Calories: 220
Fat: 9 g
Carbohydrates: 22 g
Protein: 12 g

Lunch: Bean and Vegetable Soup with Bread

Ingredients:
- 1 can of bean and vegetable soup
- 1 slice of whole wheat bread

Instructions:
1. Heat the soup in a pot over medium heat.
2. Toast one slice of whole wheat bread.
3. Plate the soup and serve with the toast.

Nutrition Information (per serving):
Calories: 312
Fat: 4 g
Carbohydrates: 56 g
Protein: 17 g

Snack: Greek yoghurt and Almonds

Ingredients:
- 1 cup of plain Greek yoghurt
- ½ cup of almonds

Instructions:
1. Plate the Greek yoghurt and top with almonds.

Nutrition Information (per serving):
Calories: 472
Fat: 25 g
Carbohydrates: 26 g
Protein: 31 g

Dinner: Grilled Salmon with Roasted Cauliflower and Brown Rice

Ingredients:
- 4-ounce grilled salmon fillet
- 1 cup of roasted cauliflower
- ½ cup of cooked brown rice

Instructions:
1. Preheat the oven to 375°F.

2. Place the salmon on a baking sheet and bake in the preheated oven for 15-20 minutes.

3. Meanwhile, toss the cauliflower with olive oil, salt, and pepper and spread on a baking sheet.

4. Roast the cauliflower in the preheated oven for 20-25 minutes.

5. Cook the brown rice according to package instructions.

6. Plate the salmon, cauliflower, and brown rice.

Nutrition Information (per serving):

Calories: 467

Fat: 17 g

Carbohydrates: 40 g

Protein: 35 g

DAY 16

Breakfast: Overnight Oats with Banana and Walnuts

Ingredients:

- 1 cup of rolled oats
- 1 banana, sliced
- 1 tablespoon of walnuts
- 1 cup of skim milk

Optional: Honey for sweetness

Instructions:

1. In a medium-sized bowl, combine the oats, banana slices, and walnuts.

2. Pour the skim milk over the oat mixture and stir until combined.

3. Cover the bowl and place in the fridge overnight.

4. In the morning, sweeten the oats with honey if desired.

Nutrition Information (per serving):
Calories: 300
Fat: 5g
Carbohydrates: 47g
Protein: 13g

Snack: Apple and Low-Fat Cottage Cheese

Ingredients:
- 1 apple, cored and sliced
- -1½ cup low-fat cottage cheese

Instructions:
1. Prepare the apple slices and place them on a plate.
2. Place the cottage cheese on the side of the apple slices.

Nutrition Information (per serving):
Calories: 170
Fat: 2g
Carbohydrates: 28g
Protein: 15g

Lunch: Spinach Salad with Grilled Chicken

Ingredients:
- 1 cup of fresh spinach
- 1 grilled chicken breast, sliced
- 1 cup of fresh fruit

Optional: Olive oil and vinegar for dressing
Instructions:
1. Place the spinach in a medium-sized bowl.

2. Top the spinach with the grilled chicken slices and fresh fruit.

3. Drizzle olive oil and vinegar over the salad, if desired.

Nutrition Information (per serving):
Calories: 330
Fat: 12g
Carbohydrates: 20g
Protein: 36g

Snack: Plain Greek yoghurt and Almonds

Ingredients:
- 1 cup of plain Greek yoghurt
- ½ cup of almonds

Instructions:
1. Place the Greek yoghurt in a bowl.
2. Top the yoghurt with the almonds.

Nutrition Information (per serving):
Calories: 390
Fat: 23g
Carbohydrates: 18g
Protein: 26g

Dinner: Grilled Chicken Breast and Quinoa

Ingredients:
- 4-ounce grilled chicken breast
- ½ cup of cooked quinoa
- 1 cup of steamed vegetables

-Optional: Olive oil and lemon juice for dressing
Instructions:
1. Place the grilled chicken breast on a plate.
2. Top the chicken with the cooked quinoa and steamed vegetables.
3. Drizzle olive oil and lemon juice over the dish, if desired.

Nutrition Information (per serving):
Calories: 380
Fat: 9g
Carbohydrates: 36g
Protein: 33g

DAY 17
Breakfast: Banana Almond Smoothie

Ingredients:
- 1 banana
- 1 cup almond milk
- 1 scoop protein powder

Instructions:
1. Place banana, almond milk, and protein powder in a blender.
2. Blend until smooth.
3. Serve and enjoy!

Nutrition Information (per serving):
Calories: 170
Fat: 2.5g
Carbohydrates: 25g
Protein: 10g.

Snack: Hard-Boiled Egg and Toast

Ingredients:
- 1 hard-boiled egg
- 2 slices of whole wheat toast

Instructions:
1. Boil the egg for 10 minutes.
2. Toast the slices of whole wheat toast.
3. Place the egg on top of the toast.
4. Serve and enjoy!

Nutrition Information (per serving):
Calories: 306
Fat: 10.3g
Carbohydrates: 37g
Protein: 13g.

Lunch: Hummus Wrap

Ingredients:
- 2 whole-wheat tortillas
- 4 tablespoons hummus
- 1 lettuce leaf
- 1 tomato, sliced
- 1 cucumber, sliced

Instructions:
1. Spread 2 tablespoons of hummus on each tortilla.
2. Place the lettuce leaf, tomato, and cucumber slices on each tortilla.
3. Roll up the tortillas and cut in half.
4. Serve and enjoy!

Nutrition Information (per serving):
Calories: 303
Fat: 10.3g
Carbohydrates: 38g
Protein: 11g.

Snack: Greek yoghurt and Almonds

Ingredients:
- 1 cup plain Greek yoghurt
- ½ cup almonds

Instructions:
1. Place Greek yoghurt in a bowl.
2. Top with almonds.
3. Serve and enjoy!

Nutrition Information (per serving):
Calories: 437
Fat: 25.2g
Carbohydrates: 25g
Protein: 24g.

Dinner: Grilled Salmon, Roasted Cauliflower, and Brown Rice

Ingredients:
- 4 ounces grilled salmon
- 1 cup roasted cauliflower
- ½ cup cooked brown rice

Instructions:

1. Preheat the oven to 425°F.

2. Place salmon on a baking sheet and roast for 15 minutes.

3. Toss cauliflower with olive oil, salt, and pepper and roast for 15 minutes.

4. Cook brown rice according to package Instructions: .

5. Serve salmon, roasted cauliflower, and brown rice and enjoy!

Nutrition Information (per serving):

Calories: 444

Fat: 17.4g

Carbohydrates: 35g, 1

Protein: 33g.

DAY 18

Breakfast: Oatmeal with Blueberries and Walnuts

Ingredients:

- 1/2 cup old-fashioned oats
- 1 cup skim milk
- 1/4 cup fresh or frozen blueberries
- 1 tablespoon chopped walnuts

Instructions:

1.In a medium pot, bring the milk to a boil.

2. Stir in the oats and reduce the heat to medium-low.

3. Cook, stirring occasionally, for about 5 minutes or until thickened.

4. Stir in the blueberries and walnuts.

5. Serve warm.

Nutrition Information (per serving):
Calories: 258
Fat: 5.2 g
Carbohydrates: 43.8 g
Protein: 9.5 g

Snack: Apple and Low-Fat Cottage Cheese

Ingredients:
- 1 apple, cored and sliced
- ½ cup low-fat cottage cheese

Instructions:
1.In a small bowl, mix together the apple slices and cottage cheese.
2. Serve immediately.

Nutrition Information (per serving):
Calories: 143
Fat: 2.2 g
Carbohydrates: 20.1 g
Protein: 10.3 g

Lunch: Turkey and Vegetable Wrap with Hummus

Ingredients:
- 1 whole wheat tortilla
- 2 ounces sliced turkey
- 1/4 cup shredded lettuce
- 1/4 cup diced tomatoes
- 2 tablespoons hummus

Instructions:

1.Lay the tortilla on a flat surface.

2. Top with the turkey, lettuce, tomatoes, and hummus.

3. Roll up the tortilla and serve.

Nutrition Information (per serving):

Calories: 234

Fat: 5.8 g

Carbohydrates: 27.6 g

Protein: 17.9 g

Snack: Plain Greek yoghurt and Almonds

Ingredients:

- 1 cup plain Greek yoghurt
- 1/2 cup almonds

Instructions:

1. In a bowl, mix together the yoghurt and almonds.

2. Serve immediately.

Nutrition Information (per serving):

Calories: 369

Fat: 21.6 g

Carbohydrates: 18.9 g

Protein: 22.3 g

Dinner: Grilled Chicken Breast with Quinoa and Steamed Vegetables

Ingredients:

- 4-ounce grilled chicken breast

- 1/2 cup cooked quinoa
- 1 cup steamed vegetables (such as broccoli, carrots, and zucchini)

Instructions:

1. Grill the chicken breast until cooked through.

2. In a bowl, mix together the quinoa and steamed vegetables.

3. Serve the chicken with the quinoa and vegetables.

Nutrition Information (per serving):

Calories: 290

Fat: 6.3 g

Carbohydrates: 27.3 g

Protein: 30.5 g

fibre: 5.7 g

DAY 19

Breakfast: Egg White Omelet with Spinach, Mushrooms and Tomatoes

Ingredients:

- 4 egg whites
- 2 tablespoons of olive oil
- 2 cups of fresh spinach
- 1 cup of sliced mushrooms
- 1/2 cup chopped tomatoes
- Salt and pepper to taste

Instructions:

1. Heat the olive oil in a large skillet over medium heat.

2. Add the spinach and mushrooms to the skillet and cook for about 5 minutes, stirring occasionally.

3. Add the tomatoes and cook for another 2 minutes.

4. In a separate bowl, whisk the egg whites and season with salt and pepper.

5. Pour the egg whites into the skillet and stir gently to combine with the vegetables.

6. Cook until the eggs are set, about 3-4 minutes.

7. Serve with 2 slices of whole grain toast.

Nutrition Information (per serving):
Calories: 220
Protein: 15 g
Fat: 12 g
Carbohydrates: 11 g

Snack: Hard-Boiled Egg with Toast

Ingredients:
- 2 large eggs
- 2 slices of whole wheat toast
- Salt and pepper to taste

Instructions:
1. Place the eggs in a pot and cover with cold water.

2. Bring the water to a boil, then reduce the heat and simmer for 8-10 minutes.

3. Remove the eggs from the hot water and place in a bowl of ice water.

4. Toast the bread and serve with the eggs.

5. Season with salt and pepper to taste.

Nutrition Information (per serving):
Calories: 186
Protein: 10 g

Fat: 9 g
Carbohydrates: 16 g

Lunch: Grilled Vegetable Wrap with Hummus

Ingredients:
- 2 whole wheat tortillas
- 1/2 cup of hummus
- 1 cup of grilled vegetables (such as bell peppers, onions, mushrooms, and zucchini)
- Salt and pepper to taste

Instructions:
1. Preheat a grill or grill pan over medium-high heat.
2. Grill the vegetables for 4-5 minutes, flipping once.
3. Spread the hummus on the tortillas and top with the grilled vegetables.
4. Roll up the tortillas and serve with 1 cup of fresh fruit.

Nutrition Information (per serving):
Calories: 303
Protein: 12 g
Fat: 10 g
Carbohydrates: 40 g

Snack: Greek yoghurt and Almonds

Ingredients:
- 1 cup of plain Greek yoghurt
- 1/2 cup of almonds
- 1 tablespoon of honey (optional)

Instructions:
1. In a bowl, combine the Greek yoghurt and almonds.
2. Drizzle with honey, if desired.

Nutrition Information (per serving):
Calories: 474
Protein: 25 g
Fat: 27 g
Carbohydrates: 34 g

Dinner: Grilled Salmon Fillet with Roasted Cauliflower and Brown Rice

Ingredients:
- 4-ounce salmon fillet
- 1 cup of cauliflower florets
- 1 tablespoon of olive oil
- 1/2 cup of cooked brown rice
- Salt and pepper to taste

Instructions:
1. Preheat the oven to 400°F.
2. Place the cauliflower florets on a baking sheet and toss with the olive oil.
3. Roast in the oven for 20 minutes, flipping once.
4. Meanwhile, preheat a grill or grill pan over medium-high heat.
5. Season the salmon with salt and pepper and cook for 4-5 minutes on each side.
6. Serve the salmon with the roasted cauliflower and brown rice.

Nutrition Information (per serving):
Calories: 382
Protein: 30 g
Fat: 16 g
Carbohydrates: 26 g

DAY 20

Breakfast: 2 Eggs Over-Easy with Toast and Fresh Fruit

Ingredients:
- 2 eggs
- 2 slices of whole grain toast
- ½ cup of fresh fruit

Instructions:
1. Heat a non-stick skillet over medium heat.
2. Crack the eggs into the skillet and cook until the whites have set and the yolks are still runny, about 2 minutes.
3. Flip the eggs and cook for an additional 1 minute.
4. Toast the bread.
5. Serve the eggs over-easy with the toast and fresh fruit.

Nutrition Information (per serving):
Calories: 254
Fat: 9 g
Carbohydrates: 28 g
Protein: 14 g

Snack: Apple and Cottage Cheese

Ingredients:
- 1 apple

- ½ cup of low-fat cottage cheese

Instructions:

1. Cut the apple into slices.

2. Serve the apple slices with the cottage cheese.

Nutrition Information (per serving):

Calories: 109

Fat: 2 g

Carbohydrates: 12 g

Protein: 9 g

Lunch: Tuna Salad Sandwich

Ingredients:

- 1 can of tuna
- ½ cup of diced celery
- 1 tablespoon of mayonnaise
- 2 slices of whole wheat bread
- 1 cup of fresh fruit

Instructions:

1. Mix the tuna, celery and mayonnaise together in a bowl.

2. Spread the tuna salad onto one slice of the bread.

3. Top with the other slice of bread.

4. Serve with the fresh fruit.

Nutrition Information (per serving):

Calories: 371

Fat: 10 g

Carbohydrates: 39 g

Protein: 27 g

Snack: Greek yoghurt and Almonds

Ingredients:
- 1 cup of plain Greek yoghurt
- ½ cup of almonds

Instructions:
1. Place the Greek yoghurt in a bowl.
2. Top with the almonds.
3. Enjoy!

Nutrition Information (per serving):
Calories: 471
Fat: 29 g
Carbohydrates: 28 g
Protein: 25 g

Dinner: Grilled Chicken with Quinoa and Vegetables

Ingredients:
- 4-ounce grilled chicken breast
- ½ cup of cooked quinoa
- 1 cup of steamed vegetables

Instructions:
1. Preheat the grill to medium-high heat.
2. Place the chicken on the grill and cook for 4-5 minutes per side, or until cooked through.
3. Cook the quinoa according to package instructions.
4. Steam the vegetables until tender.
5. Serve the grilled chicken with the quinoa and vegetables.

Nutrition Information (per serving):
Calories: 354
Fat: 8 g
Carbohydrates: 31 g
Protein: 37 g

DAY 21
Breakfast: Overnight Oats with Banana and Walnuts

Ingredients:
- ½ cup rolled oats
- 1 banana, sliced
- 2 tablespoons chopped walnuts
- 1 cup skim milk

Dash of cinnamon (optional)

Instructions:
1. Place the oats in a jar or container.
2. Top with banana slices and walnuts.
3. Pour in the milk and stir to combine.
4. Refrigerate overnight.
5. Serve cold or warm with a dash of cinnamon.

Nutrition Information (per serving):
Calories: 288
Fat: 7g
Carbohydrates: 43g
Protein: 11g

Snack: Hard-Boiled Egg with Toast

Ingredients:
- 1 large egg
- 2 slices of whole wheat bread

Instructions:
1. Place the egg in a pot and cover with water.
2. Bring the water to a boil, then reduce the heat to low and simmer for 10 minutes.
3. Remove the egg from the pot and place in a bowl of cold water.
4. Toast the bread and then serve the egg on top of the toast.

Nutrition Information (per serving):
Calories: 225
Fat: 9g
Carbohydrates: 27g
Protein: 10g

Lunch: Bean and Vegetable Soup

Ingredients:
- 1 tablespoon olive oil
- 1 onion, chopped
- 2 cloves garlic, minced
- 1 large potato, diced
- 1 cup cooked black beans
- 2 cups vegetable broth
- ½ teaspoon dried oregano
- ½ teaspoon dried basil
- Salt and pepper to taste

Instructions:

1. Heat the olive oil in a large pot over medium heat.

2. Add the onion and garlic and cook until softened, about 5 minutes.

3. Add the potato, black beans, and vegetable broth and bring to a boil.

4. Reduce the heat to low and simmer for 15 minutes.

5. Stir in the oregano, basil, salt, and pepper.

6. Serve with a slice of whole wheat bread.

Nutrition Information (per serving):

Calories: 229

Fat: 5g

Carbohydrates: 35g

Protein: 10g

Snack: Plain Greek yoghurt with Almonds

Ingredients:

- 1 cup plain Greek yoghurt
- ½ cup almonds

Instructions:

1. Place the Greek yoghurt in a bowl.

2. Top with the almonds.

Nutrition Information (per serving):

Calories: 356

Fat: 20g

Carbohydrates: 18g

Protein: 24g

Dinner: Grilled Salmon Fillet with Roasted Cauliflower and Brown Rice

Ingredients:
- 4-ounce salmon fillet
- 1 cup cauliflower florets
- 2 tablespoons olive oil
- ½ teaspoon garlic powder
- ½ teaspoon dried oregano
- Salt and pepper to taste
- ½ cup cooked brown rice

Instructions:
1. Preheat the oven to 400°F.
2. Place the cauliflower florets on a baking sheet and drizzle with olive oil. Sprinkle with garlic powder, oregano, salt, and pepper.
3. Bake for 20 minutes, stirring halfway through.
4. Meanwhile, heat a skillet over medium-high heat. Add the salmon fillet and cook for 4 minutes per side.
5. Serve the salmon with the roasted cauliflower and cooked brown rice.

Nutrition Information (per serving):
Calories: 456
Fat: 22g
Carbohydrates: 24g
Protein: 37g

Day 22:
Breakfast: Smoothie with banana, almond milk, and protein powder.
Snack: 1 apple, ½ cup of low-fat cottage cheese.
Lunch: Spinach salad with grilled chicken, 1 cup of fresh fruit.
Snack: 1 cup of plain Greek yoghurt, ½ cup of almonds.
Dinner: 4-ounce grilled chicken breast, ½ cup of cooked quinoa, 1 cup of steamed vegetables.

Day 23:
Breakfast: Egg white omelet with spinach, mushrooms, and tomatoes, 2 slices of whole grain toast.
Snack: 1 hard-boiled egg, 2 slices of whole wheat toast.
Lunch: Hummus wrap with lettuce, tomato, and cucumber, 1 cup of fresh fruit.
Snack: 1 cup of plain Greek yoghurt, ½ cup of almonds.
Dinner: 4-ounce grilled salmon fillet, 1 cup of roasted cauliflower, ½ cup of cooked brown rice.

Day 24:
Breakfast: Oatmeal with blueberries and walnuts, 1 cup of skim milk.
Snack: 1 apple, ½ cup of low-fat cottage cheese.
Lunch: Turkey wrap with lettuce, tomato, and avocado, 1 cup of fresh fruit.
Snack: 1 cup of plain Greek yoghurt, ½ cup of almonds.
Dinner: 4-ounce grilled chicken breast, ½ cup of cooked quinoa, 1 cup of steamed vegetables.

Day 25:

Breakfast: 2 eggs over-easy, 2 slices of whole grain toast, ½ cup of fresh fruit.

Snack: 1 hard-boiled egg, 2 slices of whole wheat toast.

Lunch: Grilled vegetable wrap with hummus, 1 cup of fresh fruit.

Snack: 1 cup of plain Greek yoghurt, ½ cup of almonds.

Dinner: 4-ounce grilled salmon fillet, 1 cup of roasted cauliflower, ½ cup of cooked brown rice.

Day 26:

Breakfast: Smoothie with banana, almond milk, and protein powder.

Snack: 1 apple, ½ cup of low-fat cottage cheese.

Lunch: Tuna salad sandwich on whole wheat bread, 1 cup of fresh fruit.

Snack: 1 cup of plain Greek yoghurt, ½ cup of almonds.

Dinner: 4-ounce grilled chicken breast, ½ cup of cooked quinoa, 1 cup of steamed vegetables.

Day 27:

Breakfast: Overnight oats with banana and walnuts, 1 cup of skim milk.

Snack: 1 hard-boiled egg, 2 slices of whole wheat toast.

Lunch: Bean and vegetable soup, 1 slice of whole wheat bread.

Snack: 1 cup of plain Greek yoghurt, ½ cup of almonds.

Dinner: 4-ounce grilled salmon fillet, 1 cup of roasted cauliflower, ½ cup of cooked brown rice.

Day 28:

Breakfast: Egg white omelet with spinach, mushrooms, and tomatoes, 2 slices of whole grain toast.

Snack: 1 apple, ½ cup of low-fat cottage cheese.

Lunch: Spinach salad with grilled chicken, 1 cup of fresh fruit.

Snack: 1 cup of plain Greek yoghurt, ½ cup of almonds.

Dinner: 4-ounce grilled chicken breast, ½ cup of cooked quinoa, 1 cup of steamed vegetables.

Grocery Shopping List for WEEK 4

Produce:
- Bananas (6)
- Apples (9)
- Spinach (2 bags)
- Fresh fruit of choice (5 cups)
- Mushrooms (1 container)
- Tomatoes (4)
- Blueberries (1 cup)
- Cauliflower (1 head)
- Avocado (1)
- Lettuce (1 head)
- Cucumber (1)
- Bean and vegetable soup mix (1 package)

Dairy/Refrigerated:
- Almond milk (1 carton)
- Low-fat cottage cheese (3 cups)
- Plain Greek yoghurt (9 cups)

- Eggs (18)
- Skim milk (2 cups)

Protein:
- Chicken breast (22 ounces)
- Grilled salmon fillet (16 ounces)
- Tuna (1 can)

Pantry Items:
- Protein powder (7 scoops, if using)

Grains:
- Whole grain toast (22 slices)
- Whole wheat bread (3 slices)
- Cooked quinoa (2 cups)
- Brown rice (1 cup)
- Oatmeal (2 cups)
- Whole wheat wrap (3)
- Bread (1 loaf)
- Overnight oats (7 servings)

Nuts and Seeds:
- Walnuts (1cup)
- Almonds (3 cups)

Recipes

DAY 22

Breakfast: Smoothie with banana, almond milk, and protein powder.

Ingredients:
- 1 banana
- 1 cup of almond milk
- 1 scoop of protein powder

Instructions:
1. Place banana, almond milk and protein powder into a blender.
2. Blend until smooth.
3. Serve and enjoy!

Nutrition Information (per serving):
Calories: 210
Fat: 4g
Protein: 15g
Carbohydrates: 30g

Snack: 1 apple, ½ cup of low-fat cottage cheese.

Ingredients:
- 1 apple
- ½ cup of low-fat cottage cheese

Instructions:
1. Slice the apple into thin slices.
2. Top with the cottage cheese.
3. Enjoy!

Nutrition Information (per serving):
Calories: 153
Fat: 3g
Protein: 13g

Carbohydrates: 21g

Lunch; Spinach salad with grilled chicken, 1 cup of fresh fruit.

Ingredients:
- 2 cups of fresh spinach
- 4 ounces of grilled chicken
- 1 cup of fresh fruit

Instructions:
1. Combine the spinach, chicken and fruit in a bowl.
2. Drizzle with your favorite dressing.
3. Enjoy!

Nutrition Information (per serving):
Calories: 298
Fat: 6g
Protein: 33g
Carbohydrates: 28g

Snack: 1 cup of plain Greek yoghurt, ½ cup of almonds.

Ingredients:
- 1 cup of plain Greek yoghurt
- ½ cup of almonds

Instructions:
1. Place the yoghurt in a bowl.
2. Top the yoghurt with the almonds.
3. Enjoy!

Nutrition Information (per serving):
Calories: 441
Fat: 22g
Protein: 28g
Carbohydrates: 24g

Dinner: 4-ounce grilled chicken breast, ½ cup of cooked quinoa, 1 cup of steamed vegetables.

Ingredients:
- 4 ounces of grilled chicken breast
- ½ cup of cooked quinoa
- 1 cup of steamed vegetables

Instructions:
1. Cook the quinoa according to package instructions.
2. Grill the chicken until cooked through.
3. Steam the vegetables until tender.
4. Combine the quinoa, chicken and vegetables in a bowl.
5. Serve and enjoy!

Nutrition Information (per serving):
Calories: 302
Fat: 7g
Protein: 25g
Carbohydrates: 33g

DAY 23

Breakfast: Egg White Omelet with Spinach, Mushrooms, and Tomatoes

Ingredients:
- 3 large egg whites
- 3 ounces spinach
- 3 ounces mushrooms, chopped
- 3 ounces tomatoes, chopped
- 2 slices of whole grain toast

Instructions:
1. Heat a large non-stick skillet over medium heat.
2. Add the egg whites, spinach, mushrooms, and tomatoes to the pan.
3. Cook for 3-4 minutes, stirring occasionally, until the vegetables are softened and the eggs are cooked through.
4. Serve with two slices of whole grain toast.

Nutrition Information (per serving):
Calories: 300
Fat: 5g
Carbohydrates: 34g
Protein: 21g

Snack: Hard-Boiled Egg with Whole Wheat Toast

Ingredients:
- 1 large egg
- 2 slices of whole wheat toast

Instructions:
1. Place the egg in a pot of cold water and bring to a boil.

2. Simmer for 10 minutes.
3. Remove the egg from the pot and let cool.
4. Peel and slice the egg.
5. Serve with two slices of whole wheat toast.

Nutrition Information (per serving):
Calories: 222
Fat: 9g
Carbohydrates: 23g
Protein: 12g

Lunch: Hummus Wrap with Lettuce, Tomato, and Cucumber

Ingredients:
- 1 large whole wheat wrap
- 3 ounces hummus
- 3 ounces lettuce, shredded
- 3 ounces tomato, diced
- 3 ounces cucumber, diced
- 1 cup of fresh fruit

Instructions:
1. Spread the hummus on the wrap.
2. Top with the lettuce, tomato, and cucumber.
3. Roll up the wrap.
4. Serve with one cup of fresh fruit.

Nutrition Information (per serving):
Calories: 355
Fat: 12g
Carbohydrates: 48g

Protein: 11g

Snack: Plain Greek yoghurt with Almonds

Ingredients:
- 1 cup of plain Greek yoghurt
- ½ cup of almonds

Instructions:
1. Place the yoghurt in a bowl.
2. Top with the almonds.
3. Serve.

Nutrition Information (per serving):
Calories: 473
Fat: 25g
Carbohydrates: 34g
Protein: 21g

Dinner: Grilled Salmon Fillet, Roasted Cauliflower, and Brown Rice

Ingredients:
- 4 ounces of grilled salmon fillet
- 1 cup of roasted cauliflower
- ½ cup of cooked brown rice

Instructions:
1. Preheat the oven to 400°F.
2. Place the salmon fillet on a baking sheet.
3. Roast for 8-10 minutes, until cooked through.
4. Meanwhile, steam the cauliflower for 5 minutes.

5. Serve the salmon fillet with the roasted cauliflower and cooked brown rice.

Nutrition Information (per serving):
Calories: 472
Fat: 16g
Carbohydrates: 43g
Protein: 38g

DAY 24
Breakfast: Oatmeal with Blueberries and Walnuts

Ingredients:
- 1 cup of old-fashioned oats
- 1 cup of skim milk
- ½ cup of fresh blueberries
- 2 tablespoons of chopped walnuts

Instructions:
1. In a medium saucepan, bring the milk to a simmer over medium-high heat.
2. Stir in the oats and reduce the heat to low.
3. Cook, stirring occasionally, for about 5 minutes until the oats are soft and creamy.
4. Stir in the blueberries and walnuts.
5. Serve warm.

Nutrition Information (per serving):
Calories: 315
Fat: 10.7g
Carbohydrates: 43.9g
Protein: 11.7g

Snack: Apple and Cottage Cheese

Ingredients:

- 1 large apple, cored and sliced
- ½ cup of low-fat cottage cheese

Instructions:

1. Slice the apple and arrange on a plate.
2. Top with cottage cheese.
3. Serve.

Nutrition Information (per serving):
Calories: 187
Fat: 2.7g
Carbohydrates: 29.6g
Protein: 11.2g

Lunch: Turkey Wrap

Ingredients:

- 1 whole-wheat wrap
- 2 ounces of sliced turkey
- 2 slices of lettuce
- 1 slice of tomato
- 1 slice of avocado
- 1 tablespoon of light mayonnaise
- 1 cup of fresh fruit

Instructions:

1. Lay the wrap on a flat surface.
2. Spread the mayonnaise over the wrap.
3. Layer the lettuce, tomato, and avocado on top.

4. Add the turkey slices.

5. Roll the wrap tightly and cut in half.

6. Serve with fresh fruit.

Nutrition Information (per serving):
Calories: 398
Fat: 16.3g
Carbohydrates: 42.8g
Protein: 22.2g

Snack: Greek yoghurt and Almonds

Ingredients:
- 1 cup of plain Greek yoghurt
- ½ cup of almonds

Instructions:
1. In a bowl, combine the yoghurt and almonds.
2. Mix until combined.
3. Serve.

Nutrition Information (per serving):
Calories: 461
Fat: 28.7g
Carbohydrates: 25.1g
Protein: 22.3g

Dinner: Grilled Chicken, Quinoa, and Steamed Vegetables

Ingredients:
- 4 ounces of grilled chicken breast
- ½ cup of cooked quinoa

- 1 cup of steamed vegetables (such as broccoli, cauliflower, carrots, or green beans)

Instructions:

1. Preheat the grill to medium-high heat.

2. Grill the chicken breast for about 4 minutes per side, or until cooked through.

3. Place the cooked quinoa in a bowl.

4. Top with the steamed vegetables.

5. Slice the cooked chicken and add to the bowl.

6. Serve warm.

Nutrition Information (per serving):

Calories: 393

Fat: 10.4g

Carbohydrates: 33.2g

Protein: 34.3g

DAY 25

Breakfast: 2 Eggs Over Easy with 2 Slices of Whole Grain Toast and ½ Cup of Fresh Fruit

Ingredients:

- 2 eggs
- 2 slices of whole grain toast
- ½ cup of fresh fruit

Instructions:

1. Heat a small non-stick skillet over medium heat and add a bit of butter.

2. Crack the eggs into the skillet and cook until the whites are set and the yolks are still runny.

3. Toast the slices of whole grain toast.

4. Serve the eggs over-easy on the toast and with the fruit on the side.

Nutrition Information (per serving):
Calories: 292
Fat: 11g
Carbohydrates: 36g
Protein: 13g

Snack: Hard-Boiled Egg and 2 Slices of Whole Wheat Toast

Ingredients:
- 1 hard-boiled egg
- 2 slices of whole wheat toast

Instructions:
1. Hard-boil the egg.
2. Toast the slices of whole wheat toast.
3. Serve the hard-boiled egg with the toast.

Nutrition Information (per serving):
Calories: 166
Fat: 6g
Carbohydrates: 21g
Protein: 8g

Lunch: Grilled Vegetable Wrap with Hummus and 1 Cup of Fresh Fruit

Ingredients:
- 1 whole wheat tortilla

- 4 tablespoons of hummus
- ½ cup of grilled vegetables (such as bell peppers, onions, and mushrooms)
- 1 cup of fresh fruit

Instructions:

1. Heat a skillet over medium-high heat.
2. Add the vegetables to the skillet and cook until they are lightly browned.
3. Place the tortilla on a plate and spread the hummus on it.
4. Add the grilled vegetables to the tortilla and wrap it up.
5. Serve with the fruit on the side.

Nutrition Information (per serving):
Calories: 296
Fat: 5g
Carbohydrates: 44g
Protein: 12g

Snack: 1 Cup of Plain Greek yoghurt and ½ Cup of Almonds

Ingredients:

- 1 cup of plain Greek yoghurt
- ½ cup of almonds

Instructions:

1. Place the cup of Greek yoghurt in a bowl.
2. Top with the almonds.
3. Enjoy.

Nutrition Information (per serving):
Calories: 428

Fat: 26g

Carbohydrates: 19g

Protein: 27g

Dinner: 4-Ounce Grilled Salmon Fillet, 1 Cup of Roasted Cauliflower, and ½ Cup of Cooked Brown Rice

Ingredients:
- 4-ounce grilled salmon fillet
- 1 cup of roasted cauliflower
- ½ cup of cooked brown rice

Instructions:

1. Preheat the oven to 400°F.

2. Place the salmon fillet on a greased baking sheet.

3. Bake for 15 minutes or until the salmon is cooked through.

4. Meanwhile, roast the cauliflower by tossing it with olive oil, salt, and pepper and then roasting it in the oven for 20 minutes.

5. Cook the brown rice according to package instructions.

6. Serve the salmon with the roasted cauliflower and the cooked brown rice.

Nutrition Information (per serving):

Calories: 461

Fat: 16g

Carbohydrates: 34g

Protein: 44g

DAY 26:

Breakfast: Banana Almond Protein Smoothie

Ingredients:

- 1 banana
- 1 cup almond milk
- 1 scoop of protein powder

Instructions:

1. Place all ingredients in a blender and blend until smooth.
2. Serve immediately.

Nutrition Information (per serving):
Calories: 180
Fat: 3g
Carbohydrates: 25g
Protein: 15g

Snack: Apple and Cottage Cheese

Ingredients:

- 1 apple
- ½ cup low-fat cottage cheese

Instructions:

1. Slice the apple into wedges.
2. Serve with the cottage cheese.

Nutrition Information (per serving):
Calories: 140
Fat: 2.5g
Carbohydrates: 20g
Protein: 10g

Lunch: Tuna Salad Sandwich

Ingredients:

- 2 ounces canned tuna
- 1 tablespoon mayonnaise
- 1 tablespoon diced onion
- 1 teaspoon diced celery
- 2 slices of whole wheat bread
- 1 cup of fresh fruit

Instructions:

1. In a medium bowl, mix together tuna, mayonnaise, onion, and celery.
2. Spread the mixture onto one slice of bread.
3. Place the remaining slice of bread on top.
4. Cut the sandwich in half, if desired.
5. Serve with fresh fruit.

Nutrition Information (per serving):
Calories: 320
Fat: 10g
Carbohydrates: 38g
Protein: 20g

Snack: Plain Greek yoghurt and Almonds

Ingredients:

- 1 cup plain Greek yoghurt
- ½ cup almonds

Instructions:

1. Place the yoghurt in a bowl.
2. Top with the almonds.
3. Enjoy.

Nutrition Information (per serving):
Calories: 420
Fat: 25g
Carbohydrates: 20g
Protein: 25g

Dinner: Grilled Chicken and Quinoa

Ingredients:
- 4 ounces grilled chicken breast
- ½ cup cooked quinoa
- 1 cup steamed vegetables

Instructions:
1. Place the grilled chicken breast on a plate.
2. Top with quinoa and steamed vegetables.
3. Serve.

Nutrition Information (per serving):
Calories: 340
Fat: 7g
Carbohydrates: 33g
Protein: 35g

DAY 27:
Breakfast: Overnight Oats with Banana and Walnuts

Ingredients:
- ½ cup rolled oats
- 1 ripe banana, mashed
- 2 tablespoons chopped walnuts
- 1 cup skim milk

- 1 teaspoon honey (optional)

Instructions:

1. In a medium bowl, combine oats, mashed banana, and chopped walnuts.

2. Pour in the milk and stir until the mixture is combined.

3. Cover the bowl with plastic wrap and place in the refrigerator overnight.

4. In the morning, remove from the refrigerator and stir in honey (if desired).

5. Serve and enjoy!

Nutrition Information (per serving):

Calories: 239

Fat: 5.5 g

Carbohydrates: 41 g

Protein: 8.2 g

Snack: Hard-boiled Egg, 2 Slices of Whole Wheat Toast

Ingredients:

- 2 large eggs
- 2 slices of whole wheat bread

Instructions:

1. Place the eggs in a medium saucepan and cover with cold water.

2. Place the saucepan over high heat and bring the water to a boil.

3. Once the water is boiling, reduce the heat to medium-low and let the eggs cook for 10 minutes.

4. After 10 minutes, remove the eggs from the pan and place in a bowl of cold water.

5. Once the eggs are cool enough to handle, peel them and slice in half.

6. Toast the slices of whole wheat bread.

7. Serve the eggs with the toast and enjoy!

Nutrition Information (per serving):
Calories: 305
Fat: 10.8 g
Carbohydrates: 35.4 g
Protein: 15.6 g

Lunch: Bean and Vegetable Soup, 1 Slice of Whole Wheat Bread

Ingredients:
- 1 tablespoon olive oil
- 1 onion, chopped
- 2 cloves garlic, minced
- 1 teaspoon dried oregano
- 1 teaspoon ground cumin
- 1 can (14.5 ounces) diced tomatoes
- 1 can (15 ounces) black beans, drained and rinsed
- 4 cups vegetable broth
- 1 cup diced carrots
- 1 cup diced celery
- 1 cup diced zucchini
- 1 teaspoon salt
- ¼ teaspoon black pepper
- 1 slice of whole wheat bread

Instructions:
1. Heat the olive oil in a large pot over medium heat.

2. Add the onion, garlic, oregano, and cumin and cook until the onion is translucent, about 5 minutes.

3. Add the tomatoes, black beans, vegetable broth, carrots, celery, and zucchini and bring to a boil.

4. Reduce the heat and let the soup simmer for 20 minutes.

5. Add the salt and pepper and stir.

6. Serve the soup with the slice of bread and enjoy!

Nutrition Information (per serving):

Calories: 286

Fat: 6.3 g

Carbohydrates: 44.5 g

Protein: 11.5 g

Snack: 1 Cup of Plain Greek yoghurt, ½ Cup of Almonds

Ingredients:

- 1 cup plain Greek yoghurt
- ½ cup almonds

Instructions:

1. Scoop the yoghurt into a bowl.

2. Sprinkle the almonds on top of the yoghurt.

3. Serve and enjoy!

Nutrition Information (per serving):

Calories: 462

Fat: 29.7 g

Carbohydrates: 29.7 g

Protein: 18.3 g

Dinner: 4-ounce Grilled Salmon Fillet, 1 Cup of Roasted Cauliflower, ½ Cup of Cooked Brown Rice

Ingredients:
- 4-ounce salmon fillet
- 1 tablespoon olive oil
- Salt and pepper, to taste
- 1 cup cauliflower florets
- 1 tablespoon olive oil
- ½ teaspoon garlic powder
- ½ teaspoon paprika
- ½ cup cooked brown rice

Instructions:

1. Preheat the oven to 400°F.

2. Place the salmon fillet on a baking sheet lined with parchment paper and brush with olive oil. Sprinkle with salt and pepper.

3. In a separate bowl, combine the cauliflower florets, olive oil, garlic powder, and paprika.

4. Spread the cauliflower mixture onto a separate baking sheet lined with parchment paper.

5. Place both baking sheets in the oven and bake for 15 minutes.

6. Remove the baking sheets from the oven and serve the salmon and cauliflower with the cooked brown rice.

Nutrition Information (per serving):
Calories: 437
Fat: 15.7 g
Carbohydrates: 38.7 g
Protein: 29.6 g

DAY 28

Breakfast: Egg White Omelet with Spinach, Mushrooms, and Tomatoes

Ingredients:
- 2 eggs, whites only
- 2 tablespoons spinach, chopped
- 2 mushrooms, sliced
- 2 cherry tomatoes, sliced
- 2 slices of whole grain toast

Instructions:
1. Heat a small non-stick pan over medium heat.
2. In a bowl, whisk together the egg whites until frothy.
3. Add the spinach, mushrooms, and tomatoes to the pan and cook for 2-3 minutes, stirring occasionally.
4. Pour the egg whites over the vegetables and cook until the eggs are set, about 3-4 minutes.
5. Flip the omelet and cook for another minute.
6. Serve with the toast.

Nutrition Information (per serving):
Calories: 289
Fat: 5g
Protein: 20g
Carbohydrates: 37g

Snack: Apple with Low-Fat Cottage Cheese

Ingredients:
- 1 apple, sliced

- ½ cup low-fat cottage cheese

Instructions:

1. Slice the apple and place on a plate.
2. Top with cottage cheese.

Nutrition Information (per serving):
Calories: 160
Fat: 2g
Protein: 11g
Carbohydrates: 28g

Lunch: Spinach Salad with Grilled Chicken

Ingredients:
- 1 cup fresh spinach leaves
- 2 tablespoons balsamic vinegar
- 2 tablespoons olive oil
- 2 tablespoons feta cheese, crumbled
- 2 tablespoons slivered almonds
- 4 ounces grilled chicken, diced
- 1 cup fresh fruit (optional)

Instructions:

1. In a large bowl, combine the spinach, vinegar, oil, feta cheese, and almonds.
2. Add the grilled chicken and mix until everything is evenly combined.
3. Serve with fresh fruit, if desired.

Nutrition Information (per serving):
Calories: 298
Fat: 17g

Protein: 25g
Carbohydrates: 13g

Snack: Plain Greek yoghurt with Almonds

Ingredients:
- 1 cup plain Greek yoghurt
- ½ cup almonds

Instructions:
1. Place the Greek yoghurt and almonds in a bowl and mix until combined.
2. Serve.

Nutrition Information (per serving):
Calories: 410
Fat: 22g
Protein: 18g
Carbohydrates: 28g

Dinner: Grilled Chicken Breast with Quinoa and Steamed Vegetables

Ingredients:
- 4 ounces grilled chicken breast
- ½ cup cooked quinoa
- 1 cup steamed vegetables

Instructions:
1. Heat a grill or grill pan over medium-high heat.
2. Grill the chicken until cooked through, about 5 minutes per side.

3. Meanwhile, cook the quinoa according to package Instructions: .

4. Steam the vegetables until tender, about 5 minutes.

5. Serve the chicken, quinoa, and vegetables together.

Nutrition Information (per serving):
Calories: 286
Fat: 8g
Protein: 28g
Carbohydrates: 24g

Chapter 4:

Breakfast Recipes

Shrimp Spring Rolls with Peanut Dipping Sauce

Preparation Time: 30 minutes
Cook Time: 5 minutes
Total Time: 35 minutes
Servings: 10 rolls

Ingredients:
Peanut dipping sauce:

- ½ cup (120 ml) hoisin sauce.
- Peanut butter: ¼ cup (60 ml)
- 1 tablespoon (15 ml) of rice vinegar, Marukan Seasoned Gourmet
- 1 tablespoon (10 g) chopped peanuts, with extra for dusting.

Shrimp Spring Rolls:

- 6 ounces (170 g) thin rice noodles Thin: 10 (265 g) jumbo shrimp
- 16-20 count 10 round rice paper wrappers
- 10 Boston lettuce leaves, thick stem ends removed and split in half.
- 1 cup (60 g) Shredded carrots
- 1 cup (75 g) of finely shredded red cabbage
- 1 cup (45 g) bean sprouts
- 20 mint leaves
- ½ cup (2 g) cilantro leaves, gently packed.

Instructions:

1. In a medium mixing bowl, combine the hoisin sauce, peanut butter, water, rice vinegar, and peanuts until smooth.
2. If you like a thinner consistency, add additional water.
3. Transfer to a serving dish and garnish with chopped peanuts.

Shrimp rolls;

1. In a medium pot, bring three quarts of water to a boil. Cook the dry rice noodles until soft but not mushy, about 4 to 6 minutes, or according to package recommendations.
2. Transfer to a colander, rinse with cold water, and chill until ready to use. Do not discard the water.
3. Boil water, add shrimp, and cook for 1-1 ½ minutes until pink and opaque.
4. Remove the prawns from the water immediately, drain and refrigerate.
5. Once cooled, remove the shell if it is still attached and cut the prawns lengthwise in half to make two pieces. Set aside.
6. Fill a pie dish or big bowl with enough chilly water to contain the rice paper.
7. Place a moist dish towel on the cutting board. Immerse one rice paper sheet in water for 15-20 seconds.
8. Remove, shake off excess water, and place flat on the moist towel. The paper may still appear rigid, but it will become malleable as you make each roll.

9. Place one piece of lettuce on the bottom third of the rice paper. On the lettuce, arrange 2 to 3 tablespoons of noodles, 1 tablespoon of carrots, 1 tablespoon of cabbage, and a few bean sprouts.
10. Roll the paper halfway into a cylinder. Fold the sides into an envelope design.
11. Place two prawn halves, cut side down, along the crease. Place some cilantro and mint leaves next to the prawns. Continue rolling the paper into a tight cylinder to seal.
12. Repeat with the remaining wrappers. Store with the seam side down. Serve immediately with peanut dipping sauce.

Nutritional Information:
Calories: 357
Carbohydrates: 35g
Protein: 5g
Fat: 2g

Blueberry Kale Smoothie

Preparation Time: 5 Minutes
Total Time: 5 Minutes
Servings: 1

Ingredients:
- 1 cup milk. Almond, soy, rice, coconut, or cow milk is acceptable.
- 1 cup kale, chopped and rinsed

- 1 banana.
- 1.5 cups blueberries, fresh or frozen.
- 1 tablespoon honey.

Instructions:
1. Blend all of the ingredients together until its smooth, then pour it into a glass and serve.

Nutritional Information:
Calories: 477
Carbohydrates: 94g
Protein: 14g
Fat: 10g

Overnight Oats with Chia Seeds and Fresh Fruits

Preparation Time: 5 minutes
Refrigeration Time: 8 hours
Total Time (including refrigeration time)* : 8 hours 5 minutes
Servings: 6

Ingredients:
- ½ cup rolled oats
- 2 tablespoons chia seeds
- 2 tablespoons blueberries
- 2 tablespoons blackberries
- ½ cup almond milk
- ¼ cup water, and 1 mashed banana.

- Ground cinnamon, ¼ tsp (optional).

Instructions:
1. Choose an airtight container or jar. Add all ingredients except the berries. Stir thoroughly.
2. Refrigerate for at least eight hours.
3. In the morning, add the berries and enjoy.

Nutritional Information:
Calories: 246
Carbohydrates: 44g
Protein: 6.5g
Fat: 6g

Greek yoghurt Parfait with Nuts and Maple Syrup

Preparation Time: 10 minutes
Total Time: 10 minutes
Servings: 4

Ingredients:
- ⅓ cup granola
- ⅓ cup Greek yoghurt
- 1 tbsp chopped almonds
- 1 tbsp chopped cashews
- ½ cup mixed berries
- 1 tbsp maple syrup.

Instructions:
1. Add a layer of yoghurt to your glass.
2. Add a layer of granola.
3. Add some nuts, berries, and syrup as a third layer.
4. Repeat this procedure until you've used everything.

Nutritional Information:

Calories: 444

Carbohydrates: 60g

Protein: 14g

Fat: 17g

Avocado Toast on Whole Grain Bread

Preparation Time: 5 minutes

Total Time: 5 minutes

Servings: 4

Ingredients:
- 2 slices whole-grain bread
- 1 ripe avocado
- A sprinkle of salt.

Instructions:
1. Toast the bread pieces.
2. Dice open the avocado and spoon out the flesh.
3. Mash until smooth, then add a touch of salt.
4. Spread the mashed avocado evenly on each slice of bread.

Nutritional Information:

Calories: 474

Carbohydrates: 42.8g

Protein: 12.2g

Fat: 31.6g

Scrambled Eggs with Spinach and Olive Oil

Preparation Time: 30 minutes

Total Time: 30 minutes

Servings: 6

Ingredients:
- Three huge eggs.
- 3 oz baby spinach
- ½ tbsp olive oil
- 1 ½ tbsp skim milk and 1/16 tsp salt (or to taste).
- Black pepper, 1/16 tsp, or to taste

Instructions:
1. Place oil in a pan over medium-high heat.
2. Crack the eggs into a bowl and beat them. Combine skim milk, salt, and pepper.
3. Pour into the pan and whisk continually.
4. Add the spinach as it begins to firm and cook until it wilts.

Nutritional Information:

Calories: 117
Carbohydrates: 2g
Protein: 10.5g
Fat: 14g

Protein Powder and Frozen Fruit Plant-Based Smoothie

Preparation Time: 5 minutes
Total Time: 5 minutes
Servings: 2

Ingredients:

- 1 ½ cups frozen mixed berries
- 1 cup of unsweetened soy milk
- 1 whole banana, and one scoop vanilla plant-based protein powder.

Instructions:

1. Blend all the ingredients in a blender until smooth.

Nutritional Information:

Calories: 439
Carbohydrates: 64g
Protein: 31g
Fat: 8g

Whole Wheat Pancakes with Fresh Ginger and Soy Sauce

Preparation Time: 45 minutes
Total Time: 45 minutes
Servings: 6

Ingredients:

- To make pancakes, combine ½ cup whole wheat flour, 1/16 tsp salt, and 3 tbsp thinly sliced scallions.
- ¼ cup hot water, 1 tablespoon sesame seed oil.
- To make dipping sauce, combine soy sauce, rice wine vinegar, grated ginger, sugar, and optional red pepper flakes (1/16 tsp).

Instructions:

1. Mix the ingrdeints for the dipping sauce in a bowl, .Set aside.
2. Add the flour to a food processor. Begin by carefully pouring in hot water until the dough forms a ball.
3. Dust a surface with flour and knead until smooth.
4. Place in a bowl and cover for 30 minutes.
5. Divide the dough into four equal pieces.
6. Flatten each with a rolling pin. Glaze with sesame seed oil and garnish with scallions.
7. Roll each into a log, then coil into a tight spiral. Flatten into a disc.
8. Fry the dough until browned on both sides.

Nutritional Information:

Calories: 113

Carbohydrates: 14g

Protein: 2.5g

Fat: 5.5g

Smoked Salmon on Whole Wheat Toast

Preparation Time: 30 minutes

Total Time: 30 minutes

Servings: 5

Ingredients:

- 1/2 a whole wheat baguette
- 1 oz smoked salmon
- 4 tbsp cream cheese
- ¼ tbsp lemon juice, and ¼ tsp lemon zest

Instructions:

1. Slice your baguette in half and toast.
2. In a bowl, combine the cream cheese, lemon juice, and lemon zest.
3. Spread over each baguette half.
4. Layer the salmon pieces and seal the sandwich.

Nutritional Information:

Calories: 324

Carbohydrates: 42g

Protein: 26g

Fat: 4g

Peanut Butter and Banana Oatmeal

Preparation Time: 15 minutes
Total Time: 15 minutes
Servings: 4

Ingredients:
- ½ cup rolled oats 1 full, sliced banana
- 1 tbsp peanut butter
- ½ tbsp chia seeds
- ½ tbsp ground cinnamon
- ½ tsp salt (a touch or to taste)
- Water, 1 ½ cups

Instructions:
1. In a saucepan, combine the oats, chia seeds, salt, cinnamon, and banana slices. Add water and stir.
2. Place over medium-high heat for 10 minutes, or until the water is absorbed. Stir frequently.
3. Serve in a bowl with peanut butter and stir.

Nutritional Information:
Calories: 369
Carbohydrates: 61g
Protein: 11g
Fat: 12g

Preparation Time: 5 minutes
Refrigeration Time: 8 hours
Total Time (including refrigeration time)* 8 hours 5 minutes
Servings:

Ingredients:
- 2 ½ tbsp chia seeds
- ½ cup almond milk
- 2 tbsp strawberries
- 2 tbsp blueberries
- 2 tbsp raspberries, and ½ tbsp honey.

Instructions:
1. Combine all ingredients in an airtight jar.
2. Refrigerate for at least eight hours.
3. Enjoy chilly.

Nutritional Information:
Calories: 292
Carbohydrates: 38g
Protein: 14g
Fat: 9g

Cottage Cheese and Vegetable Frittata

Preparation Time: 35 minutes
Oven Time: 35 minutes

Total Time: 1 hours 10 minutes
Servings: 8

Ingredients (for 8 slices):
- 4 eggs
- ½ cup cottage cheese
- 1 tbsp avocado oil
- 1 diced red bell pepper
- ½ diced onion
- 1 cup chopped broccoli
- ½ cup shredded cheddar cheese
- 1 tsp salt, and ½ tsp black pepper.

Instructions:
1. Preheat the oven to 350°F (180°C).
2. In a bowl, combine the eggs, cottage cheese, salt, and pepper.
3. Put oil in a pan over medium-high heat.
4. Add the veggies and simmer until soft.
5. Add the veggies and cheddar to the egg mixture. Stir thoroughly.
6. Pour into an oven-safe pan and bake for 30 minutes.

Nutritional Information:
Calories: 134
Carbohydrates: 3.6g
Protein: 11.2g
Fat: 8.2g

Preparation Time: 30 minutes
Total Time: 30 minutes
Servings: 4

Ingredients

- 2 tablespoons olive oil.
- 12 ounces of young potatoes, thinly sliced
- 4 cups thinly sliced veggies, such as mushrooms, bell peppers, and/or zucchini (14 ounces)
- 3 thinly sliced scallions, with green and white sections separated.
- 1 teaspoon minced fresh herbs, such rosemary or thyme.
- 6 big eggs (or 4 large eggs and 4 egg whites), lightly beaten
- 2 cups packed leafy greens, like baby spinach or baby kale (2 oz.)
- ½ teaspoon salt.

Instructions:

1. Heat the oil in a big cast-iron or nonstick pan over medium heat. Add the potatoes, cover, and simmer for approximately 8 minutes, stirring occasionally, until softened.
2. Cook uncovered, stirring occasionally, until the veggies are soft and gently browned, about 8 to 10 minutes. Stir in the herbs. Spread the veggie mixture
3. along the pan's perimeter.

4. Reduce the heat to medium-low. Place the eggs and scallion greens in the centre of the pan. Cook, stirring, until the eggs are lightly scrambled, about 2 minutes.
5. Incorporate leafy vegetables into the eggs. Remove from heat and whisk until thoroughly combined. Stir in the salt.

Nutritional Information (per serving):
Calories: 254
Fat: 14g
Carbohydrates: 20g
Protein: 12g

Chapter 5:

Smoothies Recipes

Cook Time: 10 minutes
Total Time: 10 minutes
Servings: 1

Ingredients:
- 1 banana
- 2 cups diced, ripe cantaloupe
- ½ cup nonfat or low-fat plain yoghurt
- 2 teaspoons of nonfat dry milk.
- 1 ½ teaspoons frozen orange juice concentrate.
- ½ teaspoon vanilla extract.

Instructions:
1. Place the unpeeled banana in the freezer overnight (or up to three months).
2. Remove the banana from the freezer and let it to sit for about 2 minutes to soften the peel.
3. Use a paring knife to remove the skin. (Don't worry if any fibre remains.)
4. Cut the banana into bits. Add to a blender or food processor with the cantaloupe, yoghurt, dry milk, orange juice, and vanilla. Blend until smooth.

Nutritional Information (per serving):
Calories: 364
Fat: 3g
Carbohydrates: 75g
Protein: 14g

Spinach-Avocado Smoothie

Preparation Time: 5 minutes
Total Time: 5 minutes
Servings: 1

Ingredients:
- 1 cup nonfat plain yoghurt.
- 1 cup of fresh spinach.
- 1 frozen banana and ¼ avocado.
- 2 tablespoons water, 1 teaspoon honey.

Instructions:
1. Blend the yogurt, spinach, banana, avocado, water, and honey in a blender.
2. Puree till smooth.

Nutritional Information (per serving):
Calories: 357
Fat: 8g
Carbohydrates: 58g
Protein: 18g

Vegan Smoothie Bowl

Preparation Time: 10 minutes
Total Time: 10 minutes
Servings: 1

Ingredients:
- One huge banana.
- 1 cup frozen mixed berries.
- ½ cup unsweetened soymilk or other non-dairy milk.
- ¼ cup pineapple chunks.
- ½ sliced kiwi
- 1 tablespoon sliced almonds, roasted as desired
- 1 tablespoon unsweetened coconut flakes, toasted as desired
- 1 teaspoon of chia seeds.

Instructions:
1. In a blender, combine bananas, berries, and soymilk (or almond milk).
2. Blend until smooth.
3. Pour the smoothie into a bowl, then top with pineapple, kiwi, almonds, coconut, and chia seeds.

Nutritional Information (per serving):
Calories: 338
Fat 10g
Carbohydrates: 64g
Protein: 9g

Green Smoothie

Preparation Time: 5 minutes
Total Time: 5 minutes
Servings: 1

Ingredients:
- 1 huge, ripe banana.
- 1 cup packed baby kale or roughly chopped adult kale
- 1 cup of unsweetened vanilla almond milk.
- ¼ ripe avocado
- 1 tablespoon of chia seeds.
- 2 teaspoons honey.
- 1 cup ice cubes.

Instructions:
1. Blend together the banana, kale, almond milk, avocado, chia seeds, and honey.
2. Blend on high until creamy and smooth. Add ice and mix until smooth.

Nutritional Information (per serving):
Calories: 343
Fat: 14g
Carbohydrates: 55g
Protein: 6g

Mango-Ginger Smoothie

Cook Time: 10 minutes

Total Time: 10 minutes

Servings: 1

Ingredients:

- ½ cup cooked and cooled red lentils
- 1 cup of frozen mango chunks.
- ¾ cup carrot juice
- 1 teaspoon chopped fresh ginger
- 1 teaspoon honey.
- A pinch of ground cardamom, plus more for garnish.
- Three ice cubes.

Instructions:

1. Combine lentils, mango, carrot juice, ginger, honey, cardamom, and ice cubes in a blender.
2. Blend on high for 2-3 minutes, or until extremely smooth.
3. Garnish with additional cardamom if desired.

Nutritional Information (per serving):

Calories: 352

Fat: 1g

Carbohydrates: 79g

Protein: 12g

Fruit & yoghurt Smoothie

Active Time: 10 minutes

Total Time: 10 minutes

Servings: 1

Ingredients:
- ¾ cup nonfat plain yoghurt.
- ½ cup 100% pure fruit juice.
- 1 ½ cups (6 ½ ounces) of frozen fruit, like blueberries, raspberries, pineapple, or peaches

Instructions:
1. Blend yoghurt and juice until smooth. While the machine is working, pour the fruit through the hole in the cover and puree until smooth.

Nutritional Information (per serving):
Calories: 279
Fat: 2g
Carbohydrates: 56g
Protein: 12g

Berry-Almond Smoothie Bowl

Preparation Time: 10 minutes
Total Time: 10 minutes
Servings: 1

Ingredients:
- ⅔ cup frozen raspberries
- ½ cup frozen sliced banana
- ½ cup plain unsweetened almond milk

- 5 tablespoons sliced almonds divided
- ¼ teaspoon ground cinnamon
- ⅛ teaspoon ground cardamom
- ⅛ teaspoon vanilla extract
- ¼ cup blueberries
- 1 tablespoon unsweetened coconut flakes

Instructions:

1. Blend raspberries, banana, almond milk, 3 tablespoons almonds, cinnamon, cardamom, and vanilla in a blender until smooth.
2. Pour into a bowl and top with blueberries.

Nutritional Information (per serving):

Calories: 360

Fat: 19g

Carbohydrates: 46g

Protein: 9g

Pineapple Green Smoothie

Active Time: 5 minutes

Total Time: 5 minutes

Servings: 1

Ingredients:

- ½ cup unsweetened almond milk.
- ⅓ cup nonfat plain Greek yoghurt
- 1 cup baby spinach.

- 1 cup frozen banana slices (about one medium banana
- ½ cup frozen pineapple chunks.
- 1 tablespoon of chia seeds.
- 1-2 tablespoons of pure maple syrup or honey (optional).

Instructions:

1. In a blender, combine almond milk and yoghurt, then add spinach, banana, pineapple, chia seeds, and sweetener (if using).
2. Blend until smooth.

Nutritional Information (per serving):

Calories: 297

Fat: 6g

Carbohydrates: 54g

Protein: 13g

Chocolate-Banana Protein Smoothie

Preparation Time: 5 minutes

Total Time: 5 minutes

Servings: 1

Ingredients:

- 1 frozen banana.
- ½ cup cooked red lentils.
- ½ cup nonfat milk.
- 2 tablespoons of unsweetened cocoa powder.
- 1 teaspoon of pure maple syrup.

Instructions:

1. In a blender, combine the banana, lentils, milk, chocolate, and syrup. Puree till smooth.

Nutritional Information (per serving):

Calories: 310

Fat: 2g

Carbohydrates: 64g

Protein: 15g

Strawberry Basil Lime Smoothie

Preparation Time: 10 Minutes

Total Time:10 Minutes

Ingredients:

- Ten fresh basil leaves.
- 1 can of coconut milk
- 1 ½ to 2 cups frozen strawberries (you may freeze fresh ones yourself using this technique)
- 2 tablespoons fresh lime juice
- 2 tablespoons maple syrup.

Instructions:

1. Mix all ingredients in a high-speed blender.
2. Blend until smooth. Serve immediately!

Nutritional Information (per serving):

Calories: 540.14

Fat: 42.52g

Carbohydrates: 37g
Protein: 24.75g

Chapter 6:

Poultry Recipes

Chicken Marsala

Preparation Time: 20 minutes
Cook Time: 10 minutes
Total Time: 30 minutes
Servings: 4

Ingredients:
- Four boneless, skinless chicken breast cutlets.
- 1 tiny onion.
- 1 cup of crimini or porcini mushroom slices.
- 3 tablespoons olive oil.
- ½ cup of dry Marsala wine.
- 2 tablespoons minced Italian (flat leaf). parsley
- ½ cup chicken broth (or its equivalent)
- Add salt and pepper to taste.

Instructions:
1. If desired, pound the chicken between two pieces of wax paper or plastic. Season the chicken with salt and pepper if desired.
2. Heat the oil in a pan, then add the chicken. Pan fried chicken for 5minutes on each side till golden, rotating once until done. Remove and wrap in foil to keep warm.

3. Cook until the onion is transparent and the mushrooms are tender, about 5 minutes.
4. Add the wine to the pan and simmer for 1 to 2 minutes.
5. At this step, determine how much liquid to use for chicken sauce. If you need extra, add a little broth. Taste and adjust the spices.
6. Pour the veggies and sauce over the chicken, then sprinkle with parsley.

Nutritional Information (per serving):
Calories: 255
Fat: 14g
Carbohydrates: 4g
Protein: 27g

Low-Carb Chicken Greek Bowl With Tzatziki

Preparation Time: 15minutes
Cook Time: 10 minutes
Total Time: 30 minutes
Servings: 4

Ingredients:
Greek Chicken:
- 1 pound (455 g) boneless, skinless chicken breast, cut into 1-inch (2.5-cm) cubes
- 3 tablespoons (45 millilitre) Olive oil.
- 2 tablespoons (30 ml). Lemon Juice

- 1 tablespoon (15 ml) Red wine vinegar
- 1 teaspoon (3 g) Greek seasoning
- ¼ teaspoon sea salt

Tzatziki sauce:

- 8 oz. (224 g). Full-fat plain Greek yoghurt
- ½ medium Persian cucumber, grated.
- Two grated garlic cloves.
- Zest from 1 medium lemon.
- 1 tablespoon (15 ml) Fresh lemon juice.
- 2 tablespoons (8 g) Minced fresh dill
- Use sea salt as required.
- Black pepper, as needed.

Red wine vinegar dressing:

- Combine 3 tablespoons (45 ml) olive oil,
- 1 tablespoon (15 ml) red wine vinegar, and 1 teaspoon minced fresh oregano.
- Add sea salt to taste.

Salad toppings:

- Diced Persian cucumber.
- 1 cup (150 g) cherry tomatoes, halved
- 1/2 cup (58 g) thinly sliced red onions
- 1/3 cup (33 g) pitted Kalamata olives.
- 4 oz. (112 g) crumbled feta cheese

Instructions:

- Prepare the chicken, mix together oil, lemon juice, vinegar, Greek spice, and salt in a sealable container. Marinate the chicken in the refrigerator for thirty minutes, or up to overnight.
- To create the tzatziki, combine the yoghurt, cucumber, garlic, lemon zest, lemon juice, dill, salt, and black

pepper in a medium bowl. Refrigerate the tzatziki until you're ready to serve.

- Preheat a 10-inch (25-cm) or larger cast-iron pan over medium-high heat. Add the chicken and marinade to the skillet.
- Cook the chicken for 3 to 4 minutes per side, or until browned and the internal temperature reaches 165°F (74°C).
- To create the red wine vinegar dressing, combine the oil, vinegar, oregano, and salt in a small bowl.
- To construct the bowls, split the chicken into four separate serving dishes. Garnish the chicken with cucumber, tomatoes, onion, olives, and feta cheese. Pour the red wine vinegar dressing into the bowls and top with the tzatziki immediately before serving.

Nutritional Information (per serving):
Calories: 496
Fat: 32.3 g
Carbohydrates: 12.6 g
Protein: 40.4 g

Mediterranean Chicken Recipe

Prep Time 10 minutes
Cook Time 15 minutes
Total Time 25 minutes
Servings: 4

Ingredients:

- 4 boneless and skinless chicken breasts.
- 2 tablespoons of minced garlic or garlic paste.
- Kosher salt.
- Black pepper
- 1 tablespoon dried oregano, divided.
- 2 tablespoons of extra virgin olive oil.
- ½ cup dry white wine.
- 1 huge lemon, juiced.
- ½ cup chicken broth.
- One medium red onion, coarsely chopped
- Dice 4 small tomatoes (approximately 1 ½ cups).
- ¼ cup sliced green olives.
- Handful of fresh parsley, stems trimmed and leaves cut.
- crumbled feta cheese (optional)

Instructions:

1. Preparing the chicken: Pat the chicken breasts dry. Make three small incisions down each side of the chicken breast.
2. Season the chicken: Rub the garlic on both sides of the chicken, pressing it into the incisions you created. Season both sides of the chicken breasts with salt, pepper, and ½ teaspoon dry oregano.
3. Sear the chicken. In a big cast iron pan, heat the olive oil on medium-high. Sear the chicken on both sides, then pour in the white wine and reduce by half.
4. Braise the chicken: Combine the lemon juice and the chicken broth. Add the remaining ½ tablespoon of oregano and cook on medium. Cover with a lid or

securely wrapped foil. Cook for 5 to 6 minutes on one side, then flip the chicken and cook for another 5 to 6 minutes, or until the internal temperature reaches 165°F.

5. Finish the chicken and serve. Uncover and garnish with chopped onions, tomatoes, and olives. Cover again and cook for 3 minutes. Finish with parsley and feta (if using). Enjoy!

Nutritional Information (per serving):
Calories: 413.6
Carbohydrates: 14.4g
Protein: 50.5g
Fat: 14.6g

Italian chicken cacciatore

Preparation Time: 10 minutes
Cook Time: 15 minutes
Total Time: 25 minutes
Servings: 2

Ingredients:
- uncooked chicken breasts (6 oz).
- Ingredients: 1 tbsp extra virgin olive oil, 1 dash black pepper, 1 cup chopped red onion, and 2 cups raw, entire, sliced mushrooms.
- Red bell pepper, uncooked, one medium, thinly sliced
- Dried mixed herbs, 2 teaspoons
- Crushed tomatoes (14½ oz)

- Ingredients: ½ cup of low-sodium chicken stock, 1 tablespoon of balsamic vinegar.
- Green olives, 12 (chopped)
- Fresh parsley, ¼ cup flat leaf, coarsely chopped.

Instructions:

1. Cut each chicken breast into one-inch chunks. Place on a platter. Add 1 teaspoon oil. Season and then coat.
2. Heat a medium nonstick skillet over medium-high heat. Cook the chicken for 1 minute per side, or until browned. Transfer to a plate.
3. Add the remaining oil, onion, mushrooms, bell pepper, and herbs to the skillet. Cook, stirring often, for 5 minutes, or until softened. Stir in the tomatoes and stock. Season.
4. Bring to a simmer. Take the chicken and any remaining juices back to the pan. Reduce the heat to low, cover, and simmer for 5 minutes, or until the chicken is fully cooked and has reached an internal temperature of 165°F.
5. Spoon on the balsamic vinegar. Combine the olives and parsley. Serve.

Nutritional Information (per serving):

Calories: 339
Fat: 12.8 g
Carbohydrates: 32.2 g
Protein: 28.5 g

Preparation Time: 10 minutes
Cook Time: 20 minutes
Total Time: 30 minutes
Servings: 4 servings

Ingredients:
- 2 boneless and skinless chicken breasts
- ½ teaspoon salt + more to taste
- ¼ teaspoon black pepper + more to taste
- ¼ teaspoon paprika
- ¼ teaspoon garlic powder
- ¼ teaspoon dried thyme
- 4 tbsp butter split
- 8 ounces of sliced cremini mushrooms
- ¾ cup thick cream

Instructions:
1. Cut the chicken breasts in half widthwise, creating two thinner pieces. Season both sides with salt and pepper to taste.
2. Mix ¼ teaspoon salt, ¼ teaspoon powdered black pepper, paprika, garlic powder, and dried thyme in a small bowl until well blended. Set aside.
3. Heat a heavy-bottomed skillet or Dutch oven over medium heat until it is hot.
4. Add 3 tablespoons butter and stir with a wooden spoon or tongs until thoroughly melted.

5. Arrange the chicken breasts in a single layer and sprinkle with half of the spice mixture. Cook for 4–5 minutes.

6. Cook the chicken breasts for another 3-5 minutes, or until they reach a minimum internal temperature of 165 degrees Fahrenheit.

7. Remove the chicken breasts from the pan and transfer to a dish. Set aside.

8. Remove the skillet from the heat and mix in the remaining 1 tablespoon butter. Swirl and melt.

9. Add the sliced mushrooms and toss to coat with butter. Mix in the remaining seasoning combination.

10. Sauté the mushrooms for about 5 minutes, or until tender and most of the liquid has been released. If the bottom of the skillet is heavily browned, making it harder to cook the mushrooms, deglaze it with extra wine, stock, or water.

11. Pour in the heavy cream and use the bottom of a wooden spoon to scrape off any browned pieces from the pan's bottom. Once the majority of the browned pieces have been scraped away, decrease the heat to medium-low.

12. Simmer for 3-5 minutes, scraping the bottom of the skillet and stirring until the sauce thickens.

13. Remove the mushrooms and sauce from the heat, and return the chicken breasts to the pan. Spoon the sauce over them or toss to coat.

14. Garnish with parsley if preferred and serve immediately.

Nutritional Information (per serving):
Calories: 395
Carbohydrates: 4g
Protein: 27g
Fat: 30g

Curried Chicken Salad

Preparation Time: 15 minutes
Chill Time: 30 minutes
Total Time: 45 minutes
Servings: 3

Ingredients:
- ½ cup mayonnaise or plain low-fat Greek yoghurt.
- ½ teaspoon curry powder.
- ½ teaspoon cayenne pepper.
- ¼ teaspoon ground black pepper
- Poach two skinless, boneless chicken breasts (4 ounces each) and chop them into 1-inch pieces.
- 1 celery stalk, chopped.
- 1 medium red apple, chopped (do not peel).
- ½ cup chopped walnuts.
- ½ cup raisins

Instructions:
1. Mix mayonnaise or yoghurt with curry powder, cayenne pepper, and black pepper.

2. Add cubed chicken breast, celery, apples, walnuts, and raisins. Mix well to coat with the mayonnaise mixture.

3. Refrigerate for at least 30 minutes. Serve cold.

Nutritional Information (per Serving):

Calories: 352

Protein: 22g

Carbohydrates: 35g

Fat: 16g

Chicken Quesadillas

Prep Time 30 minutes

Total Time: 30 minutes

Servings: 6

Ingredients:
- ½ cup salsa.
- 1 cup tomatoes, minced
- 1 cup cilantro, minced
- 1 cup onions, minced
- 4 ounces chicken breasts, boneless and skinless
- Six parts. 8 inch whole wheat tortilla

Instructions:
1. Chop each chicken breast into bite-sized pieces.
2. Place the chicken and onions in a nonstick frying pan and heat until well cooked and tender.

3. Remove from heat and mix in the tomatoes, cilantro, and salsa.

4. To assemble, use a serving dish. Rub one part of the tortilla with water, then lay it flat and add ½ cup of chicken mixture; leave ½ inch around the rim; top with shredded cheese, and fold in half.

5. Place the chicken quesadillas in a baking sheet lined with parchment paper.

6. Lightly cover with vegetable oil and bake for up to 10 minutes, or until the quesadillas are light golden.

7. Cut in half or serve immediately as is.

Nutritional Information (per serving):
Calories: 293
Carbohydrates: 25g
Protein: 27g
Fat: 17g

Healthy Chicken Fried Rice

Preparation Time: 15minutes
Cook Time: 10minutes
Total Time: 25minutes
Servings: 8

Ingredients:
- 1 tablespoon sesame oil.
- 1 medium onion, chopped.

- Two huge eggs.
- 6 ounces cooked chicken, chopped
- 3 cups of cooked brown rice.
- 1 ½ cups frozen peas and carrots.
- 3 garlic cloves, minced
- 1 Tablespoon minced ginger
- 4 Tablespoons Soy Sauce
- Optional ingredients: 1 teaspoon rice wine vinegar.
- 1 cup fresh snap peas, halved
- 1 medium red pepper, cut thinly

Instructions:

1. Heat the olive oil in a big nonstick wok-style pan. Add the onion, peas and carrots, garlic and ginger, red pepper, and snap peas (if using).
2. Sauté the peas and carrots for 5-7 minutes, or until well cooked.
3. Add the chicken and stir to mix. Add the rice, stir to incorporate, and cook well.
4. Make a hole in the pan by spreading out the rice, chicken, and vegetables. Add the eggs and heat until scrambled. Mix the fried eggs into the rest of the dish.
5. Combine the soy sauce and rice wine vinegar. Stir to mix. You can add extra soy sauce as needed.

Nutritional Information (per serving):

Calories: 147

Fat: 3g

Carbohydrates 19g

Protein 9g

Chapter 7:

Seafood recipes

Easy Seafood Paella

Preparation Time: 20 minutes
Cook Time: 40 minutes
Total Time: 60 minutes
Servings: 6

Ingredients:

- 4 tiny lobster tails (6-12 ounces each)
- Water
- 3 tablespoons extra virgin olive oil
- Dice one big yellow onion
- soak two cups of Spanish or medium-grain rice in water for 20 minutes before draining.
- Chop 4 garlic cloves.
- Soak 2 huge pinches of Spanish saffron threads in ½ cup water.
- 1 teaspoon sweet Spanish paprika.
- 1 teaspoon cayenne pepper.
- ½ teaspoon of chilli pepper flakes (I used Aleppo pepper)
- Salt
- 2 coarsely chopped Roma tomatoes,

- 6 oz French green beans and 1 pound peeled and deveined prawns or big shrimp of your choosing.
- ¼ cup chopped fresh parsley.

Instructions:
1. Heat 3 cups of water in a big saucepan until it boils. Add the lobster tails and cook for 1-2 minutes, or until pink.
2. Turn off the heat. Use tongs to remove the lobster tails. Do not discard the lobster cooking water. Once the lobster has cooled enough to handle, remove the shell and chop into big bits.
3. In a big deep pan or cast iron skillet, heat 3 tablespoons olive oil. Increase the heat to medium-high and add the chopped onions. Saute the onions for 2 minutes, then add the rice and simmer for another 3 minutes, stirring often.
4. Now, add the chopped garlic and lobster cooking water. Add the saffron and its soaking liquid, paprika, cayenne pepper, aleppo pepper, and salt. Mix in the diced tomatoes and green beans. Bring to a boil, then decrease the liquid slightly. Cover (with a lid or securely wrapped foil) and simmer on low heat for 20 minutes.
5. Uncover the rice and press the prawns into it slightly. Add water as required. Cover and simmer for a further 10 minutes, or until the shrimp is pink. Finally, combine the cooked lobster bits. When the lobster has warmed through, turn off the heat. Garnish with parsley.
6. Serve the paella hot with your preferred white wine.

Nutritional Information (per serving):
Calories:516
Fat: 21.6g
Carbohydrates: 61.5g
Protein: 41.1g

Greek Panko Crusted Cod

Preparation Time: 5 minutes
Cook Time: 12 minutes
Total Time: 17 minutes

Servings: 4

Ingredients:
- 4 cod fillets, fresh or frozen.
- 1 cup Japanese panko breadcrumbs, gluten-free or standard.
- 2 tbsp fresh parsley finely chopped
- 1 tablespoon of dried oregano.
- 1 clove garlic, minced
- ½ lemon juice and zest.
- 1 tablespoon extra-virgin olive oil.
- Salt and pepper to taste.

Instructions:
1. Preheat the oven to 400 degrees Fahrenheit.
2. If using frozen fish, ensure that it has been thawed to room temperature.

3. Line a baking sheet with parchment or silicone mat.
4. In a small bowl, mix the panko, parsley, oregano, garlic, and lemon zest.
5. Place the fillets on the prepared baking sheet and sprinkle with olive oil, lemon juice, and salt and pepper. Flip the fillets over and repeat on the opposite side.
6. Top each fillet with the panko mixture, evenly spreading it across all four and pushing it down to firm up the fish.
7. Place the fish in the oven and bake for 12-15 minutes, or until thoroughly cooked and flaky, and the panko topping is golden brown.
8. Serve immediately with a slice of lemon.

Nutritional Information (per serving):

Calories: 262

Carbohydrates: 13g

Protein: 37g

Fat: 7g

Mediterranean Baked Halibut

Preparation Time: 5 minutes

Cook Time: 15 minutes

Total Time: 20 minutes

Servings: 2

Ingredients:
- 1 pound fresh halibut
- 2-3 tablespoons chopped sundried tomatoes.
- 2–3 tablespoons mayonnaise
- Mince 2 garlic cloves and add ¼ teaspoon dry oregano.

Optional: A dash of red pepper flakes.
- Combine 1 tablespoon fresh basil, olive oil, kosher salt, and fresh pepper to taste.

Instructions:
1. Preheat oven to 425 degrees Fahrenheit. Combine the chopped sun-dried tomatoes, mayonnaise, garlic, oregano, and red pepper flakes (if using).
2. Coat a small baking sheet with olive oil before placing the fish on top, skin side down. Sprinkle a little amount of kosher salt on the fish. Spread the mayonnaise/tomato mixture on top of the fish.
3. Bake at 425 degrees for 15 to 17 minutes. My fish was approximately 1 ½" thick and took 15 minutes. Remove from the oven and top with freshly chopped basil. Enjoy!

Nutritional Information (per serving):
Calories: 320
Carbohydrates: 4g
Protein: 43g
Fat: 14g

Creamy Coconut Indonesian Fish Curry - Kari Ikan

Preparation Time: 15 minutes
Cook Time: 15 Minutes
Total Time: 30 Minutes
Servings: 2

Ingredients:

- 400 g white fish, cut into 5 cm / 2 inch pieces
- 1 lemongrass stalk cut in half and bruised.
- 6 Thai makrut or kaffir lime leaves, entire
- 1 cup water.
- 1 cup coconut cream substitutes coconut milk.
- 3 tablespoons vegetable oil.
- Spice Paste (don't worry, it's really easy)
- 6 cloves garlic, coarsely diced.
- 3 huge red chillies, deseeded and diced (for taste).
- 2-3 tiny shallots, coarsely chopped.
- 1 tomato, chopped
- 3 tablespoons fish sauce.
- 1 tablespoon turmeric powder.
- 2 tsp ginger, chopped or minced
- 2 teaspoons of coarsely sliced lemongrass
- 2 teaspoons palm sugar
- 1 teaspoon ground coriander.
- 1 teaspoon lime juice or tamarind paste.
- ¼ teaspoon of black pepper
- 1 sprinkle of nutmeg.

Optional:

- 1–3 tiny red chillies for heat (to taste)
- White rice for serving.
- Crispy fried shallots as garnish

Instructions:

1. For the Spice Paste:

- Put everything on the spice paste list (garlic, big red chillies, tiny shallots, tomato, fish sauce, tumeric powder, ginger, lemongrass, palm sugar, crushed coriander, lime juice or tamarind paste, black pepper, nutmeg, and optional small red chilies) in a food processor or blender.
- Pulse for 30 seconds to 1 minute to create a fragrant paste.

   Ingredients:

   6 cloves garlic, 3 big red chillies, 2-3 tiny shallots, 1 tomato, 3 tbsp fish sauce, 1 tbsp turmeric powder, 2 tsp ginger, 2 tsp lemongrass, 2 tsp palm sugar, 1 tsp powdered coriander, 1 tsp lime juice, ¼ tsp black pepper, 1 pinch nutmeg, and 1 - 3 little red chillies.

2. For Curry

   Heat the vegetable oil in a big wok over medium heat. Stir in the lemongrass stem and kaffir lime leaves and cook for 1 minute. Then, add the spice paste and stir well, cooking until aromatic (1-2 minutes).

1 lemongrass stalk, 3 tablespoons vegetable oil, and 6 Thai makrut/kaffir lime leaves. Add your white fish pieces, coat with the paste, and cook for an additional minute. 400 gramme white fish

3. Next, add your water and bring to a boil. Cook for 3-5 minutes, or until the fish is fully cooked and turns from translucent to white. 1 cup water.

4. Finally, reduce the heat to medium and stir in the coconut cream. Continue to simmer for another 5 minutes, then remove from the heat. 1 cup coconut cream.

5. Serve over your preferred fluffy white rice for the greatest curry experience, then top with fried shallots.

Nutritional Information (per serving):
Calories: 897
Carbohydrates: 35g
Protein: 50g
Fat: 67g

Fish Tacos with Lime-Cilantro Slaw

Preparation Time: 10 minutes
Cook Time: 10 minutes
Servings: 6

Ingredients:
- 2 Tbsp fresh lime juice
- 2 teaspoons of chilli powder.

- 1 ½ pounds cod fillets.
- Freshly grated zest from one lime
- 2 tbsp fresh lime juice
- 2 tablespoons of light mayonnaise.
- 1 (12-ounce) bag of coleslaw mix.
- 2 Roma plum tomatoes, seeded and diced into ½-inch cubes.
- 2 scallions, white and green, coarsely chopped
- 2 tablespoons of freshly chopped fresh cilantro.
- ½ teaspoon kosher salt.
- Olive oil in a pump sprayer.
- 12 (6-inch) flour tortillas warmed
- Lime wedges for serving.

Instructions:

1. In a shallow baking dish, combine lime juice and chilli powder. Add the cod and coat it. Cover and refrigerate while preparing the slaw.
2. In a large mixing bowl, combine the lime zest, juice, and mayonnaise. Combine the coleslaw mix, tomatoes, scallions, cilantro, and salt. Set aside.
3. Spray a big nonstick pan with oil and place it over medium-high heat. Remove the fish from the baking dish, allowing the excess liquid to drain back into the dish. Cook, stirring periodically, until opaque when flaked in the thickest section with the tip of a knife, which should take approximately 8 minutes. Transfer to a serving basin and break up into big bits with a fork.

4. For each dish, spread some fish and slaw onto a tortilla, fold it, and eat it with a squeeze of lime juice, if desired.

Nutrition Information (per serving):
Calories: 247
Protein: 24g
Carbohydrates: 29g
Fat: 4g

Easy and Healthy Shrimp Scampi

Preparation Time: 10 Minutes
Cook Time: 10 Minutes
Total Time: 20 Minutes
Servings: 4

Ingredients:
- 1 tablespoon olive oil.
- 1 ½ pound medium or big prawns, peeled and deveined. Season with kosher salt and pepper as desired.
- 4 cloves garlic, chopped
- 1 small onion, finely diced
- ¼ teaspoon chilli flakes, or to taste.
- Combine 1 medium lemon zest and ½ cup fish or veggie stock.
- 2 tablespoons minced fresh parsley

Instructions:

1. Heat the oil in a big skillet over medium heat.
2. Add the prawns and drizzle with salt and pepper. Cook the prawns until pink and opaque, then put aside.
3. In the same skillet, sauté the garlic and onion for 2-3 minutes. Combine the chilli flakes, lemon juice, zest, and stock.
4. Allow the sauce to bubble for one minute. Return the prawns to the sauce and mix in the fresh parsley. Remove from heat and serve.

Nutritional Information (per serving):

Calories: 197

Carbohydrates: 6g

Protein: 35g

Fat: 4g

Provençal Baked Fish with Mushrooms & Roasted Potatoes

Preparation Time: 15 minutes

Additional Time: 45 minutes

Total Time: 1 hr

Servings: 4

Ingredients:

- Cubed Yukon Gold or red potatoes

- Trimmed and sliced fresh mushrooms (e.g., shiitake, cremini, oyster, etc.)
- 2 tablespoons extra virgin olive oil,
- ¼ teaspoon salt, and ¼ teaspoon ground pepper.
- 2 garlic cloves, peeled and sliced
- 14 ounces of halibut, grouper, or cod fillet, divided into four parts
- 4 teaspoons of lemon juice.
- 1 teaspoon Herbs de Provence
- Fresh thyme to garnish

Instructions:

1. Preheat oven to 425 degrees Fahrenheit.
2. In a large mixing bowl, combine the potatoes, mushrooms, 1 tablespoon of oil, salt, and pepper. Transfer to a 9-by-13-inch baking dish.
3. Roast the veggies for 30 to 40 minutes, or until just tender.
4. Stir the veggies, then add the garlic. Place the fish on top. Drizzle with lemon juice and the remaining 1 tablespoon oil.
5. Sprinkle with herbs de Provence. Bake for 10-15 minutes, or until the salmon is opaque in the centre and easily flaked. Garnish with thyme if desired.

Nutritional Information (per serving):

Calories: 276

Fat: 9g

Carbohydrates: 25g

Protein: 24g

20-Minute Low Carb Salmon Dinner

Prepartion Time: 15 minutes
Cook Time: 30 minutes
Total Time: 45 minutes
Servings: 4

Ingredients:

- 1 pint of baby tomatoes
- 3 cloves of garlic
- 2 tbsp olive oil, crushed red pepper to taste.
- 4 4-ounce salmon fillets, room temperature.
- Add sea salt to taste.
- 1 lemon and black pepper (to taste)
- 1 tbsp butter.
- 5 ounces of fresh baby spinach.

Instructions:

1. Preheat the oven to broil (about 500 degrees). Mince garlic cloves and cut tomatoes in half, then set aside.
2. In a large oven-safe skillet, heat olive oil over medium-high heat for about one minute. Cook garlic, tomatoes, and crushed red pepper in a pan until the tomatoes break down and the garlic turns fragrant (approximately three minutes).
3. While the tomatoes and garlic simmer, season the salmon with sea salt, black pepper, and lemon juice.
4. Push the tomatoes to the edges of the pan, leaving a space in the centre. Allow butter to melt in the centre of the pan for around 45 seconds.

5. Add the salmon to the pan with the melted butter and heat until the edges begin to turn opaque (approximately 3 minutes).

6. Place the pan in the preheated oven and roast for about eight minutes, or until the salmon is opaque and cooked through and the tomatoes have blistered. For safe ingestion, the salmon's interior temperature should be 145 degrees.

7. If you don't have a meat thermometer and are unsure, use a knife to cut one fillet in the centre. It should flake readily and remain opaque.

8. Serve the salmon and tomatoes on a bed of fresh spinach.

Nutritional Information (per serving):

Calories: 369

Carbohydrates: 9g

Protein: 36g

Fat: 21g

Healthy Mediterranean Baked Fish

Cook Time: 30 minutes

Total Time: 30 minutes

Servings: 4

Ingredients:

- 1 tablespoon of olive oil.
- 3 garlic cloves, minced

- 28 ounces of canned crushed tomatoes
- Add ¼ cup chopped fresh basil or 1 teaspoon dried. Season with salt and pepper to taste (or Mrs. Dash).
- 16-ounce white fish fillets
- 4 oz kalamata olives (or your preferred type of olive)
- 1 tablespoon of capers
- 1 lemon cut thinly

Instructions:

1. Preheat the oven to 190 degrees C (375 degrees F).
2. In a frying pan, heat olive oil and cook garlic until aromatic. Add the smashed tomatoes, basil, and salt and pepper to taste. Place the fresh basil tomato sauce in an oven-proof dish or skillet. Place the fish on top of the fresh basil tomato sauce. Place thinly sliced lemons on top of the fish fillets. Place the drained olives and capers on top of the fish and tomatoes. If desired, sprinkle a little olive oil over the top before baking.
3. Bake your healthy Mediterranean fish uncovered for 15-25 minutes, or until it flakes easily with a fork. (The time in the oven varies on the size and thickness of the fish.) Garnish with fresh basil and enjoy!

Nutritional Information (per serving):
Calories: 229
Carbohydrates: 12g
Protein: 25g
Fat: 10g

Active Time: 25 minutes
Total Time: 25 minutes
Servings: 4

Ingredients:
- 3 tablespoons extra-virgin olive oil, split 6 medium cloves garlic, sliced 1 pound spinach ¼ teaspoon salt
- 1/8 teaspoon, divided
- 1 tablespoon of lemon juice.
- 1 pound peeled and deveined shrimp (21-30 count) with ¼ teaspoon crushed red pepper.
- 1 tablespoon of freshly chopped fresh parsley.
- 1 ½ teaspoon lemon zest.

Instructions:
1. In a large saucepan, heat one tablespoon of oil over medium heat. Add half of the garlic and sauté for 1 to 2 minutes, until it begins to brown. Toss in spinach and ¼ teaspoon salt until well coated.
2. Cook, stirring once or twice, until mostly wilted, about 3 to 5 minutes. Remove from the heat and mix in the lemon juice. Put in a bowl to keep warm.
3. Increase the heat to medium-high and add the remaining 2 tablespoons of oil to the saucepan. Add the remaining garlic and sauté for 1 to 2 minutes, until it begins to brown.

4. Add the shrimp, crushed red pepper, and the remaining 1/8 teaspoon salt; simmer, tossing, until the shrimp are just cooked through, 3 to 5 minutes longer.
5. Sprinkle the prawns with lemon zest and parsley before serving over spinach.

Nutritional Information (per serving):
Calories: 226
Fat: 12g
Carbohydrates: 6g
Protein: 26g

Chapter 8:

Salad Recipes

DASH Diet Rainbow Slaw

Preparation Time: 10 minutes
Total Time: 10 minutes
Servings: 6

Ingredients:
- tablespoons mayonnaise.
- 2 tablespoons nonfat, plain Greek yoghurt
- 2 teaspoons honey
- 1 tablespoon rice vinegar.
- ¾ teaspoon celery salt.
- 14 ounces coleslaw mix
- 1 cup cherry tomatoes, halved
- 1 medium yellow bell pepper, diced.
- ¼ cup finely chopped red onion
- ¼ cup chopped fresh parsley.

Instructions:
1. In a medium bowl, combine the mayonnaise, yoghurt, honey, rice vinegar, and celery salt. Whisk until well blended.

2. Combine the coleslaw mix, tomatoes, pepper, onion, and parsley. Gently toss until the dressing is equally spread.

3. Serve or keep in refrigerator for up to three days

Nutritional information (Per servings):

Calories: 78

Carbohydrates: 10g

Protein: 2g

Fat: 4g

Low Carb Taco Salad

Preparation Time:10 minutes

Cook Time: 8-10 minutes

Total Time: 18 minutes

Servings: 6

Ingredients:

- One head of iceberg lettuce, chopped
- 3 Roma tomatoes.
- 1 bunch of onions, chopped
- 1 pound of lean ground beef (93% to 96% lean, fat drained)
- 1 pack of Mrs Dash Low-Sodium Taco Seasoning
- 12 tablespoons of sharp cheddar cheese.
- Optional toppings.
- Catalina French Dressing (Optional) (I would use the recommended portion for serving)

- ½ cup low sodium black beans (optional)
- ½ cup low sodium corn (optional)

Instructions:
1. Brown the ground beef and remove any remaining grease. Mix in the seasoning spice packet and ¾ cup water. Let the meat boil until it thickens.
2. While the meat browns, chop the salad, tomatoes, and scallions, and prepare the remaining ingredients.
3. Top the salad with cheese and dressing. Beans and maize are optional and not included in the nutritional information.

Nutritional Information (per serving):
Calories: 283
Fat: 14.7g
Carbohydrates: 14.1g
Protein: 6.3

Sesame Chicken Salad

Preparation Time: 20 minutes
Cook Time: 15 minutes
Refrigerate: 1 hour
Total Time: 1hour 35 minutes
Servings: 4

Ingredients:
- One head of iceberg lettuce, chopped

- 3 Roma tomatoes.
- 1 bunch of onions, chopped
- 1 pound of lean ground beef (93% to 96% lean, fat drained)
- 1 pack of Mrs Dash Low-Sodium Taco Seasoning
- 12 tablespoons of sharp cheddar cheese.
- Optional toppings.
- Catalina French Dressing (Optional) (I would use the recommended portion for serving)
- ½ cup low sodium black beans (optional)
- ½ cup low sodium corn (optional)

Instructions:

1. Brown the ground beef and remove any remaining grease. Mix in the seasoning spice packet and ¾ cup water. Let the meat boil until it thickens.
2. While the meat browns, chop the salad, tomatoes, and scallions, and prepare the remaining ingredients.
3. Top the salad with cheese and dressing. Beans and maize are optional and not included in the nutritional information.

Nutritional Information (per serving):

Calories: 810

Carbohydrates: 62g

Protein: 37g

Fat: 48g

Simple Greek Salad (Paleo, Gluten-Free)

Preparation Time:15 minutes
Total Time: 15 minutes
Servings: 6

Ingredients:
- 1 big, diced cucumber.
- 3 Roma tomatoes, diced
- ¼ red onion, thinly sliced
- 1 bunch parsley, chopped
- 2 ounces broccoli sprouts
- ¼ cup Kalamata olives pitted and chopped
- ¼ cup crumbled full-fat feta cheese (optional)
- 1 lemon juice. Use only 2 tablespoons olive oil, sea salt, and black pepper.

Instructions:
In a large bowl, combine cucumber, tomato, onion, parsley, broccoli sprouts, olives, feta, lemon juice, olive oil, salt, and pepper. Stir well to mix.

Nutritional Information (per serving):
Calories: 90
Fat: 7g
Carbohydrates: 5g
Protein: 2g

Preparation Time: 10 minutes
Cook Time: 10 minutes
Total Time: 20 minutes
Servings: 4

Ingredients:

- 1 pound of turkey, 1 medium onion diced, and 4 minced garlic cloves.
- 1 ½ tablespoons chilli powder.
- 2 teaspoons cumin, ½ teaspoon salt, and ½ can green chilies.
- 14-ounce can of crushed tomatoes
- One tiny lime juiced
- Add ½ tbsp brown sugar to lettuce. I used one head of lettuce.
- 1 medium tomato, chopped.
- ½ cup cheese, shredded
- 1 big avocado, chopped.
- ½ cup salsa.

Instructions:

1. How to prepare the meat:
2. In a nonstick skillet, heat the olive oil. Combine the turkey, onion, and garlic. Cook until the turkey is nearly cooked through.
3.

4. Combine the chilli powder, cumin, salt, green chilies, and smashed tomatoes. Bring the pan to a boil and cook for 8 minutes, or until the turkey is well cooked.
5. Mix in the lime juice and brown sugar. Remove from heat.
6.
7. To prepare the salad: While the meat is boiling, rinse the lettuce and arrange on a platter. Combine the tomatoes, cheese (if using), avocado, and salsa.
8. Finally, add the meat combination, and serve immediately.

Nutritional Information (per serving):
Calories: 328
Fat: 15g
Carbohydrates: 19g
Protein: 33g

Asian Chicken Salad Lettuce Wraps

Preparation Time:20 minutes
Total Time: 20 minutes
Servings: 6

Ingredients:
Salad:
- Cut 1 lb of cooked chicken into cubes and refrigerate (use leftovers or rotisserie chicken).
- 1 ½ cups broccoli slaw (may replace cabbage)

- Dice ½ medium red bell pepper and toast ¼ cup slivered or sliced almonds.
- Chop 2 green onions and dice ½ medium avocado (optional).
- Romaine or butter? Wash the lettuce and pat it dry.
- Cilantro as garnish
- Lime wedges
- Sesame seeds

Dressing:
- Orange juice (approximately 3 tablespoons).
- ½ teaspoon orange zest, 3 tablespoons coconut aminos.
- 2 tablespoons tahini, sunflower seed butter, or almond butter.
- 1 tablespoon avocado or olive oil
- 2 teaspoons toasted sesame oil
- 1 teaspoon of rice vinegar.
- 1 garlic clove, minced (or ½ teaspoon garlic powder)
- ½ tsp freshly grated ginger (or ¼ tsp powdered dry ginger)
- Add salt and pepper to taste.

Instructions:
1. In a large bowl, combine chicken, broccoli slaw, red peppers, almonds, and green onions. Set aside.
2. Prepare the dressing. Combine the ingredients in a small bowl and whisk until smooth.
3. Pour dressing over salad and toss until chicken and vegetables are evenly covered.
4. Fold in the chopped avocado, if using.

5. Serve with lettuce, fresh cilantro, and lime wedges.
   Sprinkle with sesame seeds, black and white.

Nutrition Information (per serving)
Calories: 410
Fat: 24g
Carbohydrate: 20g
Protein: 33g

Healthy Couscous Salad

Preparation Time: 7minutes
Cook Time: 10minutes
Total Time: 17minutes
Servings: 2

Ingredients:
Salad:
- 1 cup dried pearl couscous.
- One teaspoon of extra virgin olive oil
- 1 cup grape tomatoes, halved
- ½ cup cucumber, chopped
- 1 small onion, chopped.
- 10–15 fresh basil leaves
- ⅔ cup chickpeas.
- 1/3 cup crumbled feta cheese.
- 4–6 Kalamata olives

Dressing:
- 3 tablespoons extra virgin olive oil.

- 1 tablespoon red wine vinegar.
- ½ lemon juiced (should give around 1-1.5 tablespoons)
- 1 teaspoon Dijon mustard.
- ½ teaspoon of dried oregano.
- Mince 1 garlic clove and season with sea salt and black pepper.

Instructions:

1. To make the dressing, combine all of the ingredients in a bowl. Whisk well and leave aside.
2. In a saucepan, heat the oil. Add the couscous. Sauté for 2–3 minutes, until aromatic.
3. Bring the water and couscous to a boil. Cover and cook for 7-10 minutes, until soft.
4. Remove from heat, place in a fine-mesh strainer, and rinse. Shake off the excess water and put aside.
5. Combine the grape tomatoes, cucumber, olives, onion, chickpeas, basil leaves, and feta cheese in a large mixing basin. Drizzle in half of the dressing and mix thoroughly. Add more dressing to taste.
6. Add the couscous and gently combine.
7. Divide into two salad bowls and serve.

Nutritional Information (per serving):

Calories: 750
Carbohydrates: 96g
Protein: 22g
Fat: 32g

Preparation Time: 40 minutes
Cook Time: 15 minutes
Total Time: 55 minutes
Servings: 2

Ingredients:
- ¼ cup extra virgin olive oil.
- 3 teaspoons of balsamic vinegar.
- 2 teaspoons honey.
- ½ teaspoon of kosher salt.
- ¼ teaspoon of ground black pepper.
- 2 small chicken breasts, approximately 6 ounces each, lightly pounded to an equal thickness
- 6 cups fresh spinach, loosely packed.
- ⅔ cup blackberries (halved if big)
- ¼ small red onion, thinly sliced
- 1 small avocado, peeled, pitted, and cut into wedges or pieces.
- ¼ cup crumbled feta cheese.
- 3 tablespoons of freshly cut fresh basil.
- 3 tablespoons toasted pecan halves, coarsely chopped.

Instructions:
1. In a small bowl or large measuring cup, mix together the olive oil, balsamic vinegar, honey, salt, and pepper until well combined.
2. Place the chicken breasts in a shallow dish or big zip-top bag, and drizzle with half of the balsamic

mixture. Cover the dish (or seal the bag) and chill for at least 30 minutes, or up to 2 hours. Set aside the remaining half of the (unused) balsamic mixture for serving.

3. Heat an indoor grill pan or a standard nonstick pan on medium-high. Remove the chicken breasts from the marinade and shake off the excess.

4. Remove the used marinade. Once the grill pan is hot, lay the chicken breasts in it and cook for three minutes.

5. Turn and cook for 3 minutes on the other side. Flip the chicken back to the first side and decrease the heat to medium.

6. Cook the chicken for a further 9 to 10 minutes, flipping once or twice, until it is well cooked and has reached an internal temperature of 165 degrees Fahrenheit. The actual cooking time will vary according to the thickness of your chicken. Transfer to a platter, cover with foil to keep warm, and rest for 5 minutes. Cut into bite-sized pieces or longer slices as desired.

7. To Serve: Combine the spinach, blackberries, and onion in a large serving dish. Drizzle with the remaining dressing and toss to coat. Add the avocado and chicken, then top with the feta, basil, and pecans. Enjoy right now.

Nutritional Information (per serving):
Calories: 542
Carbohydrates: 18g
Protein: 47g

Fat: 32g

Simple Greek Salad (Paleo, Gluten-Free)

Preparation Time: 15 minutes
Total Time: 15 minutes
Servings 6

Ingredients:
- 1 big, diced cucumber.
- 3 Roma tomatoes, diced
- ¼ red onion, thinly sliced
- 1 bunch parsley, chopped
- 2 ounces broccoli sprouts
- ¼ cup Kalamata olives pitted and chopped
- ¼ cup crumbled full-fat feta cheese (optional)
- 1 lemon juice. Use only 2 tablespoons olive oil, sea salt, and black pepper.

Instructions:
1. In a large bowl, combine cucumber, tomato, onion, parsley, broccoli sprouts, olives, feta, lemon juice, olive oil, salt, and pepper.
2. Stir well to mix.

Nutritional Information (per serving):
Calories: 90
Fat 7g
Carbohydrates: 5g

Protein: 2g

Mediterranean Black Eyed Pea Salad

Preparation Time: 15 minutes
Total Time: 15 minutes
Servings: 6 people

Ingredients:
- 15 oz black eyed peas, washed and rinsed 6 oz grape tomatoes, chopped 1 English cucumber, trimmed and chopped ½ cup pomegranate arils (arils from ½ pomegranate).
- Chop 2 green onions, 20 mint leaves, and feta cheese (optional).

Dressing:
- 2 tablespoons pomegranate molasses.
- Juice from ½ lemon
- 4 tablespoons extra virgin olive oil.
- 1 garlic clove, minced
- Kosher salt and black pepper.

Instructions:
1. In a large mixing bowl, add black-eyed peas, diced tomatoes, cucumbers, pomegranate arils, onions, and fresh mint.
2. Make a dressing. In a small bowl, combine the pomegranate molasses (or balsamic reduction), lemon

juice, olive oil, garlic and a generous pinch of salt and pepper.

3. Pour the dressing over the black-eyed pea salad. Mix well to mix. Finish with a sprinkling of feta cheese if desired.

Nutritional Information (per serving):

Calories: 190

Carbohydrates: 25.6g

Protein: 6.5g

Fat: 7.7g

Quinoa Salad with Cherries

Preparation Time: 10 minutes

Cook Time: 15 minutes

Servings 4

Ingredients:

- 1 cup uncooked quinoa.
- ¾ cups water,
- 1 teaspoon kosher salt, and 2 tablespoons olive oil.
- Juice and zest from one lemon
- ½ cup dried cherries.
- ½ cup of roasted pine nuts.
- ¼ cup chopped scallions (white and green sections)

Instructions:

1. In a medium saucepan over medium heat, combine the quinoa and salt. Add water. Bring to a boil and lower to a simmer. Cover and cook for 10-15 minutes.
2. Remove the pot from the heat and let it settle for 2 minutes. Remove the cover and fluff with a fork before transferring to a dish.
3. Combine the olive oil, lemon juice and zest, cherries, pine nuts, and scallions. Toss thoroughly to blend.
4. Serve either room temperature or chilled.Store in the refrigerator for up to a week.

Nutritional Information (per serving):

Calories: 328

Carbohydrates: 42g

Protein: 7g

Fat: 17g

DASH Diet Southwestern Bean and Pepper Salad

Preparation Time: 10 minutes

Refrigerator Time: 30 minutes

Total Time: 40 minutes

Servings: 4

Ingredients:

- One 15-ounce can of pinto beans, drained and rinsed
- Two bell peppers, cored and diced

- Ingredients: 1 cup fresh or frozen corn kernels, thawed. Drizzle with salt and ground pepper to taste.
- 2 limes, juiced.
- 1 tablespoon olive oil.
- 1 avocado, chopped.

Instructions:
1. In a large bowl, add the beans, peppers, corn, salt and pepper.
2. Squeeze fresh lime juice to taste, then whisk with olive oil.
3. Allow the mixture to stand in the refrigerator for 30 minutes.
4. Add avocado immediately before serving.

Nutrition Information (per serving):
Calories: 245
Fat: 11g
Carbohydrates: 32g
protein: 8g

Chapter 9:

Soup Recipes

Spanish White Bean & Spinach Soup

Preparation Time: 5 minutes
Cook Time: 25 minutes
Servings: 2

Ingredients:

- 2 tablespoons extra virgin olive oil. 30 ml
- 1 tiny onion.
- 4 cloves garlic
- ½ teaspoon sweet smoked Spanish paprika. 1.15 grams ½ teaspoon dried thyme.45 g.
- 2 ½ cups canned white beans. 400 g
- 3 cups vegetable broth, 710 ml
- ¼ teaspoon saffron threads.17 g.
- 1 cup fresh spinach, 50 g
- ¼ cup finely shredded Manchego cheese. Ingredients: 30 g, sprinkle of sea salt, and a dash of black pepper

Instructions:
1. Heat a stockpot over medium heat and add 2 tablespoons extra virgin olive oil.
2. Meanwhile, finely dice one small onion and coarsely cut four cloves of garlic.

3. Add the onion and garlic into the stock pot with the olive oil, mix continuously, after 3 minutes and the onion is translucent, add in ½ tsp sweet smoked Spanish paprika and ½ tsp dried thyme, quickly mix together, then add in 2 ½ cups of canned white beans (drained and rinsed), season with sea salt and black pepper, gently mix together.

4. Once everything is properly combined, pour in 3 glasses of vegetable broth and pinch in ¼ tsp saffron threads, increase to a high heat, and mix.

5. When the soup reaches a boil, cover the stockpot and reduce the heat to low-medium.

6. After 15 minutes, remove the cover, add 1 cup fresh spinach (roughly chopped), and stir together until wilted, about 30 seconds. Then remove the stock pot from the heat.

7. Transfer the soup to shallow bowls, grate a kiss of Manchego cheese on top, and sprinkle with finely chopped parsley before serving. Enjoy!

Nutritional Information (per serving):
Calories: 492
Fat: 18g
Carbohydrates: 61g
Protein: 24g

Low sodium french onion soup with melted cheese

Low sodium french onion soup with melted cheese

Preparation Time: 15 minutes
Cook Time: 1 hour 50 minutes
Total Time: 2 hours 5 minutes
Servings: 6

Ingredients:
- 4 big onions, peeled and sliced.
- ½ teaspoon brown sugar (optional)
- 6 tablespoons butter, no salt added.
- 8 cups of no-salt beef broth or two 32-ounce cartons
- 1/3 cup of dry white table wine.
- ½ tsp powdered dried thyme
- Two bay leaves.
- ½ teaspoon pepper.

Ezoic:
- 2 tablespoons Lea and Perrins reduced sodium Worcestershire sauce.
- 1 teaspoon liquid smoke.
- 1 teaspoon of garlic powder.
- 2 tsp Herb Ox beef bouillon without sodium granules.
- 1 teaspoon Kitchen Bouquet's Browning and Seasoning Sauce
- 2 cups shredded Swiss and Gruyere cheese

Instructions:

1. Slice onions ¼ thick. Cook onions in melted butter in a large pan over medium-low heat, stirring periodically, until brown, 45 to 50 minutes.
2. Add the sautéed onions and the remaining ingredients, save the cheese, to a bigger saucepan.
3. Bring to a boil, then decrease heat and simmer for an hour. After simmering, remove the bay leaf and discard.
4. While the soup simmers, slice low-sodium bread and brush with olive oil.
5. Broil for 2 minutes per side or until golden, right before the soup is done. Optionally, the cheese can be immediately melted onto the bread.
6. Ladle soup into oven-safe bowls. Divide cheese (about ¼ cup) over bowls or bread and broil until brown and bubbling.

Nutritional Information (per serving):
Calories: 295
Carbohydrates: 11.1g
Fat: 21.3g
Protein: 17.2g

Easy Mediterranean Chickpea Soup Recipe

Preparation Time: 10minutes
Cook Time: 40minutes
Total Time: 50minutes

Servings: 6

Ingredients:
- Extra Virgin Olive Oil.
- 1 small sweet potato, peeled and chopped into little pieces
- One big yellow onion, diced
- Chop 2 celery stalks and peel and cut 2 carrots into rounds.
- Core and cut one red bell pepper and season with kosher salt.
- 3 garlic cloves, minced
- 1 tablespoon grated fresh ginger (more or less to your preference)
- 2 15-ounce cans of chickpeas, drained and rinsed
- 1 teaspoon of coriander.
- 1 teaspoon cumin.
- ¾ teaspoon turmeric.
- Dash red pepper flakes; I used Aleppo pepper.
- 1 15-ounce can of crushed tomatoes.
- 6 cups veggie broth.
- Juice of one or two limes
- 1 cup packed, chopped fresh parsley

Instructions:
1. In a large Dutch oven, heat 3 tablespoons extra virgin olive oil on medium-high until shimmering but not smoking.
2. Combine the sweet potatoes, onions, celery, carrots, and bell peppers. Season with kosher salt. Cook for 7 minutes, stirring often, or until the sweet potatoes are

tender. Combine the garlic, ginger, chickpeas, and seasonings. Cook for another 5 minutes, stirring regularly.

3. Combine the crushed tomatoes and broth. Bring to a boil for 5 minutes, then lower the heat to medium-low. Cook over medium-low heat for 25 minutes, or until the flavours blend.

4. Turn off the heat. Add the lime juice, fresh cilantro or parsley, and a bit more fresh ginger. Enjoy!

Nutritional Information (per serving):

Calories: 170

Carbohydrates: 33.5g

Protein: 6.9g

Fat: 2.1g

Vegetable Weight-Loss Soup

Active Time: 45 minutes

Additional Time: 15 minutes

Total Time: 1 hr

Servings: 8

Ingredients:

- 2 tablespoons extra virgin olive oil.
- Chop 1 medium onion, 2 medium carrots, and 2 stalks celery. Cut 12 ounces of fresh green beans into ½-inch pieces.
- 2 garlic cloves, minced

- 8 cups No-salt chicken broth or low-sodium veggie broth
- 2 (15 ounce) cans of reduced sodium cannellini or equivalent white beans, washed
- 4 cups chopped kale.
- To prepare, cut 2 medium zucchini and 4 seeded Roma tomatoes.
- 2 teaspoons of red wine vinegar.¾ teaspoon salt.
- ½ teaspoon of ground pepper
- 8 tsp premade pesto

Instructions:

1. Heat the oil in a large saucepan over medium-high heat. Combine onion, carrots, celery, green beans, and garlic. Cook, stirring regularly, until the veggies start to soften, approximately 10 minutes.
2. Bring broth to a boil. Reduce the heat to a simmer and cook, stirring occasionally, until the veggies are tender, approximately 10 minutes more.
3. Combine the white beans, kale, zucchini, tomatoes, vinegar, salt and pepper. Cook until the zucchini and kale soften, approximately 10 minutes.
4. Top each dish of soup with 1 teaspoon pesto.

Nutritional Information (per serving):

Calories: 225

Fat: 8g

Carbohydrates: 28g

Protein: 13g

Cabbage Soup

Preparation Time: 5 minutes
Cook Time: 25 minutes
Total Time: 30 minutes

Ingredients:
- 1 teaspoon oil (omit if using a nonstick saucepan).
- 1 onion, chopped
- 1 ½ cups peeled and diced potatoes. 2 small potatoes (250g)
- 2 teaspoons of smoked paprika.
- 4 cups (one litre) Vegetable Stock
- 2 cups (450 mL). water
- 1 14oz/495g can of diced tomatoes.
- 2 cups (450 g) Chopped cabbage
- Large pinch of freshly ground black pepper.

Instructions:
1. Heat the oil (if using) in a large soup pot, then add the onion and sauté for 5 minutes, or until tender but not browned.
2. If using a nonstick saucepan, skip the oil and add a dash of water if the onions begin to cling.
3. Add the potatoes and simmer for a further 2 minutes, stirring often.
4. Stir in the paprika and heat for another minute before adding the stock, water, and tomatoes. Bring to a boil, then decrease heat and simmer for 10 minutes.

5. Add the chopped cabbage and pepper and cook for another 5 minutes. If required, add more seasoning to taste.
6. Divide into dishes and serve. Will keep in the refrigerator for up to 5 days.
7. To eliminate the need for oil, sauté the onion and potatoes in a nonstick soup pan.
8. Finally, stir in the cabbage and let it to wilt naturally with the heat of the broth. This will help prevent the cabbage from becoming mushy..

Nutritional Information (per serving):

Calories: 98

Carbohydrates: 22g

Protein: 3g

Fat: 1g

Lentil Soup with Sausage

Preparation Time: 10 minutes

Cook Time: 1 hour

Total Time: 1 hour 10 minutes

Servings: 8

Ingredients:
- 2 tablespoons olive oil.
- ½ pound of breakfast sausage.
- One big onion, chopped.

- Chop 1 big carrot, 2 large celery stalks, and mince 3 cloves garlic (optional).
- 2 cups lentils.
- ½ teaspoon of salt.
- 1 tablespoon black pepper
- 1 teaspoon of turmeric powder.
- 3 quarts of chicken stock, vegetable stock, or water
- Shredded cheese for topping (optional).

Instructions:
1. In a large soup pot, heat olive oil over medium heat. Add the sausage and brown, disintegrating it as it cooks. Drain, if required.
2. Combine celery, carrots, onion, and a sprinkle of salt. Stir until the veggies are slightly cooked and any browned parts have been scraped off the bottom of the saucepan.
3. Add the garlic and turmeric, and mix to cover everything.
4. Combine lentils with chicken stock or water. Bring to a boil, then decrease heat and simmer for 45 minutes to an hour, stirring regularly, until the lentils are cooked through.
5. Season with salt and pepper. Serve hot.

Nutrition Information (per serving):
Calories: 229
Fat: 13g
Carbohydrates: 17g
Protein: 12g

Preparation Time: 20 minutes
Cook Time: 60 minutes
Total Time: 1 hours 20 minutes
Servings: 10

Ingredients:
- 1 cup chopped raw onions
- (13 oz) Yukon Gold Potatoes (1 potato, around 5 oz)
- Sweet potato, medium (2"x5"), 114 g.
- 4 cups, chopped Kale
- 3.5 cup Black Beans,
- 10 cups of homemade bone beef broth
- 4 oz gaspar's chourico

Instructions:
1. Cut gaspar's Chourico into medallion slices 3/8 inch thick.
2. Saute in a Dutch oven until lightly browned over medium heat.
3. Add chopped onions, diced into ½-inch cubes (as desired).
4. Add diced Peeled Potato, diced into ½" cubes.
5. Add diced Peeled Sweet Potato, diced into ½" cubes.
6. Cook until covered with sausage grease. 5 minutes
7. Combine bone broth, kale, and black beans.
8. Bring to a boil, then reduce to a simmer for 60 minutes.
9. Pair with dutch oven baked crusty sour dough bread.

Nutritional Information (Per Serving):

Calories: 384.2
Fat: 12.0 g
Carbohydrates: 37.5 g
Protein: 32.4 g

Chapter 10:

Snack Recipes

Healthy Nachos Recipe

Preparation Time: 10 minutes
Cook Time: 8 minutes
Total Time: 18 minutes
Servings: 4

Ingredients:

- 3 whole wheat tortillas, cut into squares and triangles
- ½ tsp cayenne pepper
- ½ tsp garlic powder
- ½ cup reduced fat cheddar cheese
- 1 cup 2% fat cottage cheese
- ½ cup black beans
- ½ cup corn
- 1 cup pico de gallo
- 4 oz sliced avocado

For garnish, use ¼ cup chopped cilantro and 1 teaspoon of spicy sauce.

Instructions:
1. Preheat oven to 425 degrees Fahrenheit.
2. On a cutting board, cut tortillas into small squares, generating approximately 25 chips each wrap.
3. Coat a baking sheet thoroughly with cooking spray.

4. Lightly coat the sliced tortilla triangles with cooking spray as well.

5. Sprinkle cayenne pepper and garlic over the chips. Flip once and repeat.

6. Place the baking sheet with coated chips in the oven.

7. Bake for around 5-7 minutes, keeping an eye on it! Oven timings may vary; avoid burning them!

8. Remove the chips from the oven (turn it off) and top with ½ cup of strong cheddar cheese.

9. Place back in the oven for 1 minute to allow cheese to melt.

10. Remove the nachos and top with black beans, corn, cottage cheese, pico de gallo and avocado!

Nutritional Information (per serving):

Calories: 188

Fat: 6g

Carbohydrates: 22g

Protein: 14g

Avocado Hummus

Preparation Time: 10 minutes

Total Time: 10 minutes

Servings: 10

Ingredients:

- 1 can (15 ounces) no-salt-added chickpeas.
- One ripe avocado, halved and pitted
- 1 cup fresh cilantro leaves.

- ¼ cup tahini
- ¼ cup extra virgin olive oil.
- ¼ cup lemon juice
- 1 clove garlic.
- 1 teaspoon ground cumin.
- ½ teaspoon salt.

Instructions:
1. Drain chickpeas and save 2 tablespoons of the liquid. Add the chickpeas and conserved liquid to a food processor.
2. Combine the avocado, cilantro, tahini, oil, lemon juice, garlic, cumin, and salt. Puree till extremely smooth. Serve with vegetables, pita chips, or crudités.

Nutritional Information (per serving):
Calories: 156
Fat: 12g
Carbohydrates: 10g
Protein: 3g

Healthy Guacamole

Preparation Time: 10 minutes
Total Time: 10 minutes
Servings: 8

Ingredients:
- Three ripe avocados.

- ¼ tsp salt, ¼ cup sliced red onion.
- 1 tablespoon lime juice.
- 1 tablespoon chopped cilantro.
- 1 smashed clove garlic (optional).
- Dice one plum tomato (optional).
- A dash of cayenne pepper, optional

Instructions:

1. Cut avocados in half and remove the peel. Chop the avocados and arrange them in a medium basin. To achieve the appropriate consistency, mash them a little (or a lot) with a fork. Sprinkle with salt.
2. Add the remaining ingredients and toss to blend thoroughly. Serve alongside fries or veggie strips.

Note: If you leave guacamole out for a time, it will start to brown. To avoid this, carefully preserve the guacamole until ready to serve. Pour the mixture into an airtight container and push it down with a spoon. Pour a thin layer of water over the guacamole, then cover the container with a lid. The coating of water prevents the guacamole from becoming brown in the fridge. When you're ready to serve, drain off the water. Stir the guac and transfer it to a serving dish. (It may be kept in the fridge for up to three days.)

Nutritional Information (per serving):
Calories: 125
Carbohydrates: 7g
Protein: 2g
Fat: 11g

Cherry-Cocoa-Pistachio Energy Balls

Preparation Time: 25 minutes
Total Time: 25 minutes
Servings: 32 balls

Ingredients:
- 1 ½ cups dried cherries.
- ¾ cup shelled salted pistachios
- ½ cup almond butter.
- 3 tablespoons chocolate powder.
- 4 tablespoons of pure maple syrup.
- ½ teaspoon ground cinnamon

Instructions:
1. Blend cherries, pistachios, almond butter, cocoa powder, maple syrup, and cinnamon in a food processor. Pulse 10 to 20 times until finely chopped, then process for approximately 1 minute, scraping down the sides as needed, until the mixture is crumbly but holds together when pushed.
2. Squeeze roughly 1 tablespoon of the mixture tightly between your palms and roll into a ball. Place in a storage container. Repeat with the remaining mixture.

Nutritional Information (per serving):
Calories: 72
Fat: 4g
Carbohydrates: 9g
Protein: 2g

Chicken Caprese Quinoa

Preparation Time: 5minutes
Cook Time: 30minutes
Total Time: 35minutes
Servings: 1

Ingredients:

- 4 oz. Boneless, skinless chicken breast.
- ¼ teaspoon black pepper
- ¼ teaspoon garlic powder.
- ½ tablespoon avocado oil
- 47 g Quinoa (about ¼ cup).
- 100 g Heirloom Cherry Tomatoes, halved (approximately 1 cup)
- 30g Pearl Mozzarella Balls quartered (approximately ½ cup)
- 20 g torn spinach (about ½ cup)
- 1 pinch salt.
- 1 sprig of basil, optional.

Instructions:

1. Preheat the stove top pan to medium heat.
2. While the pan is heated, season both sides of the chicken breast with black pepper and garlic powder.
3. Once heated, add ½ tbsp avocado oil to the pan.
4. Place the chicken in the pan and cook for 2 minutes over medium heat before flipping and cooking for another 2 minutes on the other side. Both sides should begin to become golden brown, although the centre

will appear raw If not, give each side another minute; your pan was not hot enough.

5. Then, reduce the heat to low and cover the chicken with a lid.

6. Allow to cook for about 4 minutes before flipping and covering again for another 4 minutes on the other side. After 4 minutes on each side, the chicken should be done. However, this is dependent on the size of the chicken breast; the times given are for a 4 oz breast. It is usually recommended to check the internal temperature of chicken before serving.

7. While the chicken is cooking, prepare the quinoa: First, rinse the quinoa by filling a medium basin with 2 cups of cold water.

8. Place the Quinoa in a bowl and let it soak for 3-4 minutes. Then drain the water from the basin. Next, rinse the quinoa for another 30 seconds under cold water. This enables the outer shell to open. Strain the quinoa from the water; now it's time to cook it.

9. Heat a small saucepan over medium heat, then add ½ cup water and rinsed quinoa. Cover and simmer over medium-high heat for 15 minutes, or until the water has completely absorbed into the quinoa.

10. When the chicken is done cooking, remove it from the pan and save the pan with all of the fluids for later use. Cut the chicken into bite-sized pieces.

11. Once the quinoa is ready, move it to the sauté pan where the chicken was cooked. Return the stove back to medium heat.

12. Add the cherry tomatoes, spinach, and mozzarella to the pan with the quinoa. Season with a touch of salt,

stir once, and cook for 2-3 minutes. However, leaving the dish alone will allow the mozzarella balls to stay intact while melting.

13. Once cooked, gently transfer to a serving plate, attempting to keep the mozzarella balls whole. Top with the chicken and garnish with a few basil stems.

14. Alternatively, distribute out into your meal prep containers.

Nutritional Information (per serving):

Calories: 453

Fat: 18.1g

Carbohydrates: 38.3g

Protein: 37.1g

Chapter 11:

Exercise and the 28–Day Dash Diet Plan.

Apart from Healthy eating, Exercising while on the 28-Day Dash Diet Plan can be beneficial in many ways. It can help you lose weight and improve your overall health and well-being.

Why should we exercise on the Dash Diet Plan?

Help With Weight loss

First, it can help with weight loss. When you combine a healthy diet with regular physical activity, you will burn more calories and reduce your body fat percentage. Additionally, exercise can help boost your metabolism, so you can burn more calories even when you're not exercising.

Improve Overall Health

Exercising while on the Dash Diet plan can help improve your overall health. Exercise can help strengthen your muscles and bones, improve your cardiovascular health, and reduce your risk for certain diseases such as diabetes and heart disease. Exercise can also help reduce stress and increase your energy levels.

Keep You Motivated

Exercise can help you stay motivated to stay on track with the Dash Diet plan and help you reach your weight loss goals. Exercise can also help keep you motivated to maintain a healthy lifestyle.

Boost Mental Health

Finally, exercising while on the Dash Diet plan can help improve your mental health. Exercise can help reduce anxiety and depression while also improving your self-esteem and confidence. Exercise can also help you focus and concentrate better and improve your overall mood.

Sticking to an Exercise Routine

Sticking to a regular exercise routine can be challenging, especially if you have a busy lifestyle. Here are some tips for sticking to an exercise routine on the 28-Day Dash Diet Plan:

1. **Make it a priority:** Exercise should be a priority in your daily life. Schedule your workouts like you would any other appointment and stick to it.
2. **Set realistic goals:** Set achievable goals for yourself and make sure you are able to reach them. Doing this will help you stay motivated and keep you on track.
3. **Find an exercise buddy:** Having a workout buddy can help you stay accountable and motivated to stick with your routine. Find someone who has similar goals and interests as you.
4. **Change it up:** Variety is key when it comes to exercise. Mix up your routine by trying new workouts

or changing the intensity and duration. This will help you stay interested and motivated.

5. **Reward yourself:** Don't forget to reward yourself for achieving your goals. Whether it's a massage, a new outfit, or a night out with friends, it's important to celebrate your successes.

6. **Take it slow:** Don't expect to be able to do everything right away. Start slowly and gradually increase your intensity and duration. This will help you avoid injury and burnout.

7. **Make it fun:** Exercise should be fun, so find activities that you enjoy. This could be anything from dancing to running or playing a sport. Doing activities that you enjoy will make it easier to stay motivated.

Get enough rest:

The Importance of Rest Days on the 28-Day Dash Diet Plan:

Rest days are an important part of the 28-Day Dash Diet Plan. Regular rest days help you to recover from exercise, reduce your risk of injury, and improve your performance. Rest days also allow your body to repair itself, replenish energy stores, and improve your mental and emotional wellbeing.

Rest days allow you to take a break from your routine and give your body a chance to relax. When you rest, your body can focus on repairing itself and restoring energy. This helps to keep your body functioning optimally and prevents overtraining.

Rest days also help you to avoid burnout. When you take regular breaks, it gives you an opportunity to re-evaluate your goals and make sure you are on the right track. Taking a break also helps to reduce stress and improve your overall wellbeing.

Finally, rest days are important for preventing injury. When your body is overworked, it increases your risk of injury. Taking regular breaks helps your body recover and keeps you from pushing yourself too hard.

Modifying Exercises

Modifying exercises can help you to avoid injury and ensure that you are getting the most out of your workout.

When modifying exercises, it's important to start slow and gradually increase the intensity. Begin with low-impact exercises and gradually increase the intensity as your body adjusts. For example, if you are doing a cardio exercise, start with a low intensity and gradually increase the intensity as your body becomes more comfortable.

It's also important to choose exercises that are appropriate for your fitness level. If you are a beginner, start with low-impact exercises and gradually increase the intensity as you become more comfortable. If you are an advanced exerciser, choose exercises that are challenging but still within your abilities.

Lastly, make sure to use proper form when modifying exercises. Improper form can lead to injury, so make sure you are following the correct technique. If you are unsure of how to do an exercise, consult with a trainer or do some research online.

Common Exercise Mistakes to Avoid

Not warming up: Warming up is an important part of any workout. Make sure to warm up for at least five minutes to get your heart rate up and increase blood flow.

Not stretching: Stretching helps to increase flexibility and range of motion. Make sure to stretch before and after your workout to prevent injury and improve performance.

Not listening to your body: Make sure to listen to your body and adjust your workout accordingly. If you are feeling pain or discomfort, take a break and rest.

Going too hard: Pushing yourself too hard can lead to burnout and injury. Make sure to start slow and gradually increase intensity as your body adjusts.

Not drinking enough water: Staying hydrated is an important part of any exercise program. Make sure to drink enough water before, during, and after your workouts.

Not getting enough rest: Rest days are just as important as workout days. Make sure to take at least one day off each week to let your body recover and refuel.

Adapting Your Exercises

Beginners: Beginners should focus on low-impact exercises such as walking, yoga, and swimming. These activities will help you to get used to exercising without putting too much strain on your body.

Intermediate: Once you have built up a base level of fitness, you can start to add more challenging exercises such as running, lifting weights, and high-intensity interval training.

Advanced: Advanced exercisers should focus on challenging exercises that push their body to the limit. This could include plyometrics, sprinting, and circuit training.

When adapting exercises for different levels of fitness, it's important to make sure you are using proper form. Improper form can lead to injury, so make sure you are following the correct technique. If you are unsure of how to do an exercise, consult with a trainer or do some research online.

Common Exercise-Related Injuries and How to Avoid Them

Here are some common exercise-related injuries and how to avoid them:

Muscle strains: Muscle strains happen when a muscle is overstretched or torn. To avoid this, make sure to warm up before exercise and stop if you feel pain.

Joint injuries: Joint injuries can happen when a joint is overused or pushed beyond its limits. To avoid this, focus on proper form and listen to your body.

Shin splints: Shin splints are caused by overuse of the muscles and tendons in the lower legs. To avoid this, make sure to incorporate rest days into your routine and wear supportive shoes.

Stress fractures: Stress fractures happen when bones become weak and brittle due to overuse. To avoid this, make sure to increase intensity and duration gradually and take regular rest days.

Tendinitis: Tendinitis is inflammation of the tendons due to overuse. To avoid this, focus on proper form and make sure to stretch before and after exercise.

Back pain: Back pain can be caused by poor posture or weak core muscles. To avoid this, make sure to focus on form and strengthening your core muscles.

Here is a 28 Day Light Training Plan You can follow alongside the 28 day Meal plan

Day 1:
- Wake up and stretch
- 30 minutes of moderate intensity cardio (brisk walking, jogging, swimming, biking, etc.)
- Upper body strength training (push-ups, pull-ups, planks, etc.)
- 30 minutes of stretching

Day 2:
- Wake up and stretch
- 30 minutes of low intensity cardio (walking, yoga, light jogging, etc.)
- Core strength training (crunches, leg lifts, planks, etc.)
- 30 minutes of stretching

Day 3:
- Wake up and stretch
- 30 minutes of high intensity cardio (sprinting, HIIT, etc.)
- Total body strength training (squats, burpees, lunges, etc.)
- 30 minutes of stretching

Day 4:
- Wake up and stretch
- 30 minutes of low intensity cardio (walking, yoga, light jogging, etc.)
- Core strength training (crunches, leg lifts, planks, etc.)

- 30 minutes of stretching

Day 5:
- Wake up and stretch
- 30 minutes of moderate intensity cardio (brisk walking, jogging, swimming, biking, etc.)
- Upper body strength training (push-ups, pull-ups, planks, etc.)
- 30 minutes of stretching

Day 6:
- Wake up and stretch
- 30 minutes of low intensity cardio (walking, yoga, light jogging, etc.)
- Core strength training (crunches, leg lifts, planks, etc.)
- 30 minutes of stretching

Day 7:
- Rest day

Day 8-14:
Repeat the same pattern of exercise as days 1-7.

Day 15:
- Wake up and stretch
- 30 minutes of high intensity cardio (sprinting, HIIT, etc.)
- Total body strength training (squats, burpees, lunges, etc.)
- 30 minutes of stretching

Day 16-21:
Repeat the same pattern of exercise as days 1-7.

Day 22:
- Wake up and stretch
- 30 minutes of low intensity cardio (walking, yoga, light jogging, etc.)
- Core strength training (crunches, leg lifts, planks, etc.)
- 30 minutes of stretching

Day 23-28:
Repeat the same pattern of exercise as days 1-7.